MIND DIET

D1523379

Brain Health Revolution

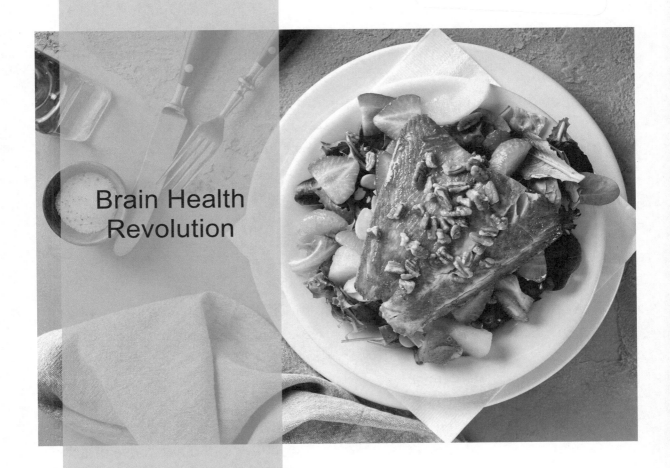

Jerry Carr

TEXT COPYRIGHT © JERRY CARR

All rights reserved. No part of this guide may be reproduced in any form without permission in writing from the publisher except in the case of brief quotations embodied in critical articles or reviews.

LEGAL & DISCLAIMER

The information contained in this book and its contents is not designed to replace or take the place of any form of medical or professional advice; and is not meant to replace the need for independent medical, financial, legal, or other professional advice or services, as may be required. The content and information in this book has been provided for educational and entertainment purposes only.

The content and information contained in this book has been compiled from sources deemed reliable, and it is accurate to the best of the Author's knowledge, information, and belief. However, the Author cannot guarantee its accuracy and validity and cannot be held liable for any errors and/or omissions. Further, changes are periodically made to this book as and when needed. Where appropriate and/or necessary, you must consult a professional (including but not limited to your doctor, attorney, financial advisor, or such other professional advisor) before using any of the suggested remedies, techniques, or information in this book.

Upon using the contents and information contained in this book, you agree to hold harmless the Author from and against any damages, costs, and expenses, including any legal fees potentially resulting from the application of any of the information provided by this book. This disclaimer applies to any loss, damages or injury caused by the use and application, whether directly or indirectly, of any advice or information presented, whether for breach of contract, tort, negligence, personal injury, criminal intent, or under any other cause of action. You agree to accept all risks of using the information presented inside this book.

You agree that by continuing to read this book, where appropriate and/or necessary, you shall consult a professional (including but not limited to your doctor, attorney, or financial advisor or such other advisor as needed) before using any of the suggested remedies, techniques, or information in this book.

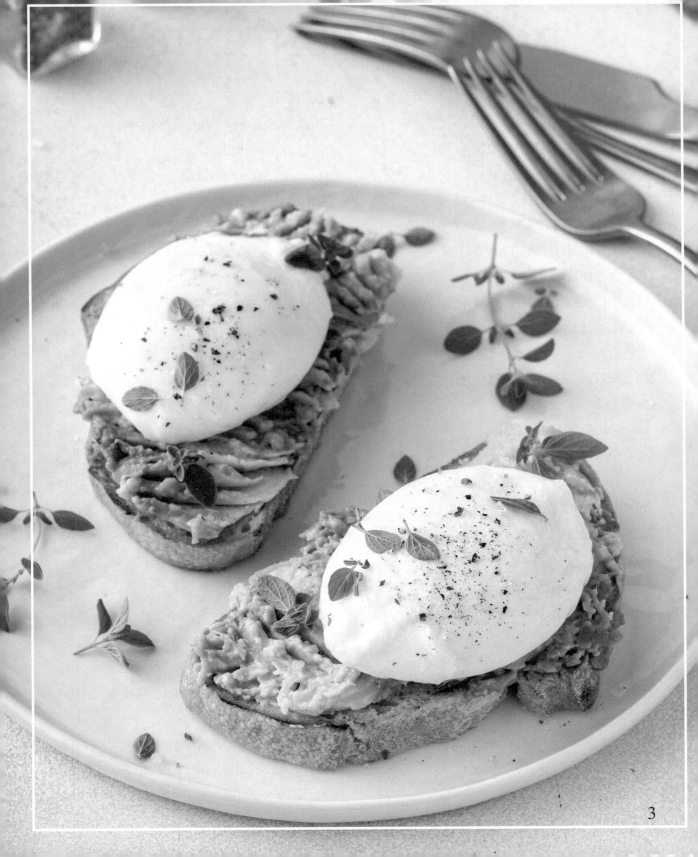

TABLE OF CONTENTS

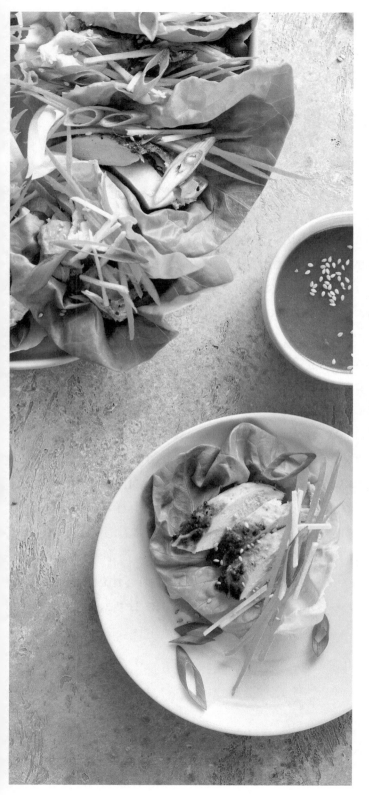

INTRODUCTION

In a world where the rapid pace of life and constant information overload have become the norm, caring for brain health is increasingly crucial. In our era where information flows endlessly, maintaining mental clarity and sharp memory becomes a paramount task. This is especially important considering the growing number of cases of Alzheimer's disease and age-related cognitive decline.

«MIND DIET: Brain Health Revolution» offers a comprehensive approach to maintaining brain health through proper nutrition and lifestyle. It is based on research demonstrating that certain foods and nutrients can help slow the aging process of the brain and reduce the risk of Alzheimer's disease.

In this book, you will find not only a variety of recipes featuring foods that positively impact the brain but also clear explanations of which specific dietary components are important for your cognitive health. We will also address lifestyle factors, including physical activity, stress management, and social interactions, which also influence brain function.

Let's explore together how to create not only healthy dishes but also a nurturing environment for your most vital organ—your brain. Welcome to the journey towards better brain health!

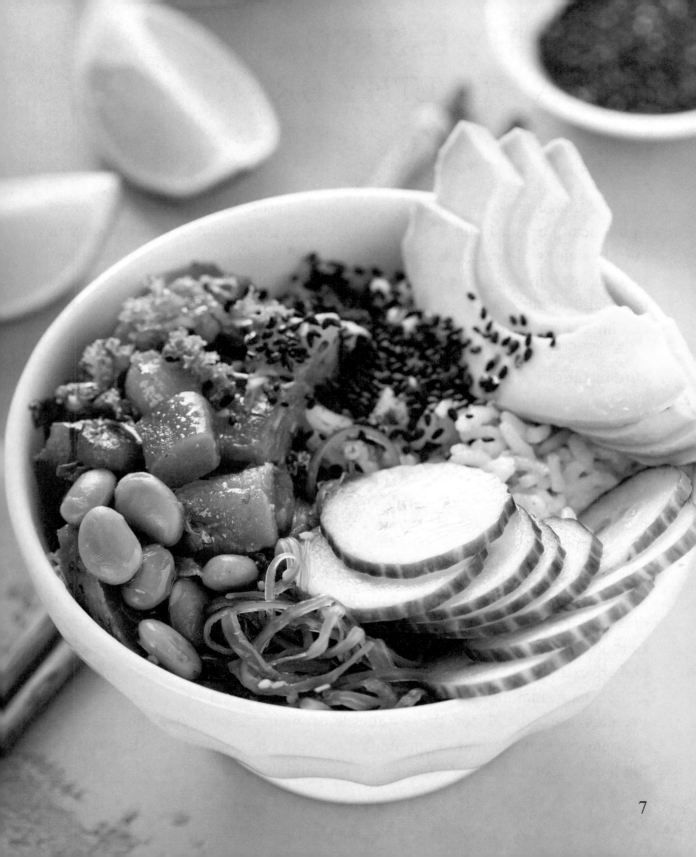

HEALTHY EATING FOR A HEALTHY BRAIN

Exploring the Link Between Diet and Brain Health

The old adage «you are what you eat» holds particularly true when it comes to the health of our brains. Our dietary choices play a crucial role not only in our physical well-being but also in the intricate workings of our brains. In this section, we will delve into the fascinating connection between what we eat and the health of our brains, examining how specific nutrients and dietary patterns can impact cognitive function, memory, and overall brain health.

Understanding the Brain's Nutritional Needs

The brain is a highly complex organ that requires a constant supply of nutrients to function optimally. While it comprises only about 2% of the body's weight, the brain consumes a disproportionate amount of energy—about 20% of the body's total energy expenditure. This energy is primarily derived from glucose, the body's primary source of fuel, which underscores the importance of maintaining stable blood sugar levels for optimal brain function.

The Role of Macronutrients in Brain Health

Macronutrients—carbohydrates, proteins, and fats—form the foundation of our diet and provide the energy and building blocks necessary for brain function. Carbohydrates, in the form of glucose, are the brain's preferred source of energy and are essential for supporting cognitive processes such as attention, memory, and decision-making.

Proteins are crucial for the synthesis of neurotransmitters, the chemical messengers that facilitate communication between brain cells. Amino acids, the building blocks of proteins, play a key role in regulating mood, cognition, and sleep.

8

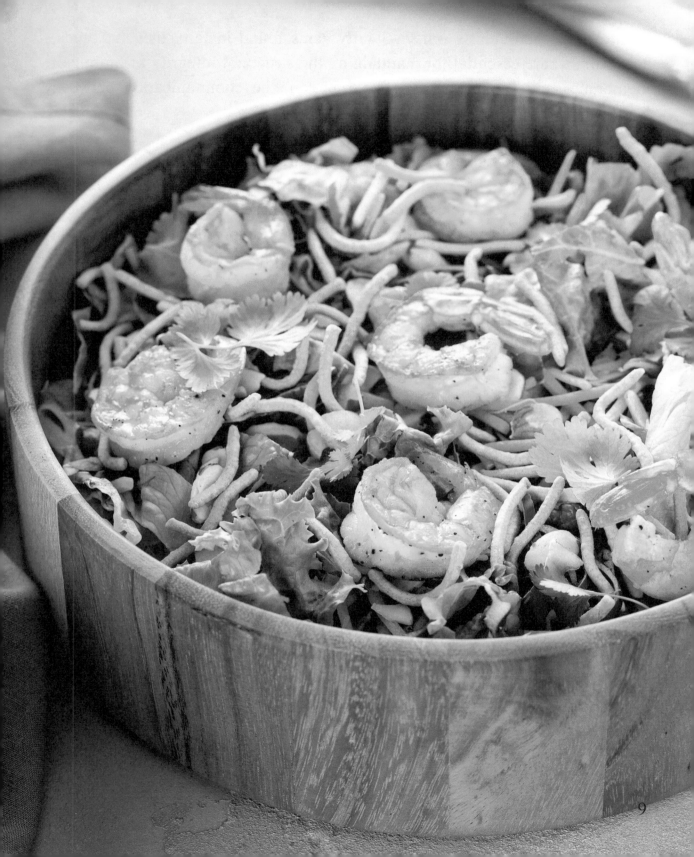

Healthy fats, particularly omega-3 fatty acids found in fatty fish, flaxseeds, and walnuts, are essential for maintaining the structural integrity of brain cell membranes and supporting synaptic function, the communication between neurons.

Antioxidants and Neuroprotective Compounds
In addition to macronutrients, a variety of micronutrients and phytochemicals found in fruits, vegetables, and other plant-based foods possess potent antioxidant and anti-inflammatory properties that help protect the brain from oxidative stress and inflammation, which are implicated in neurodegenerative diseases such as Alzheimer's and Parkinson's.

Introduction to the MIND Diet Principles: Essence and Key Guidelines

The MIND diet, which stands for Mediterranean-DASH Intervention for Neurodegenerative Delay, is a hybrid of the Mediterranean and DASH (Dietary Approaches to Stop Hypertension) diets. Developed by researchers at Rush University Medical Center in Chicago, the MIND diet is specifically designed to promote brain health and reduce the risk of Alzheimer's disease and age-related cognitive decline.

The Essence of the MIND Diet
At its core, the MIND diet emphasizes the consumption of foods that have been scientifically proven to support brain health while discouraging the intake of those associated with cognitive decline. Unlike more restrictive diets, the MIND diet offers a flexible and sustainable approach to eating, making it easier for individuals to adopt and adhere to in the long term.

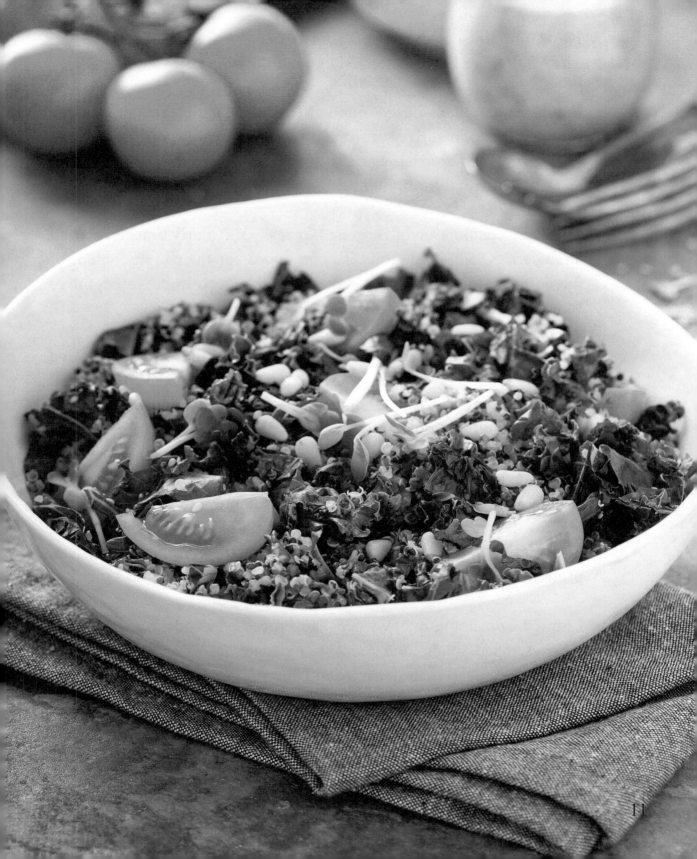

Key Guidelines of the MIND Diet

The MIND diet is characterized by the following key guidelines:

Emphasis on Plant-Based Foods: The MIND diet encourages the consumption of a variety of fruits, vegetables, whole grains, nuts, and legumes, which are rich sources of vitamins, minerals, antioxidants, and fiber essential for brain health.

Regular Consumption of Berries: Berries, particularly blueberries and strawberries, are singled out as superfoods for their high content of flavonoids, antioxidants that have been shown to improve cognitive function and protect against age-related cognitive decline.

Inclusion of Healthy Fats: Healthy fats, such as those found in olive oil, fatty fish, nuts, and seeds, are an integral part of the MIND diet. These fats provide essential omega-3 fatty acids, which support brain structure and function.

Moderate Intake of Animal Products: While not strictly vegetarian, the MIND diet recommends limiting the consumption of red meat, butter, and full-fat dairy products, which are associated with an increased risk of cognitive decline, and instead encourages the consumption of lean protein sources such as poultry and fish.

Limited Consumption of Sweets and Processed Foods: Sugary treats, pastries, fried foods, and processed snacks are discouraged on the MIND diet due to their detrimental effects on brain health and overall well-being.

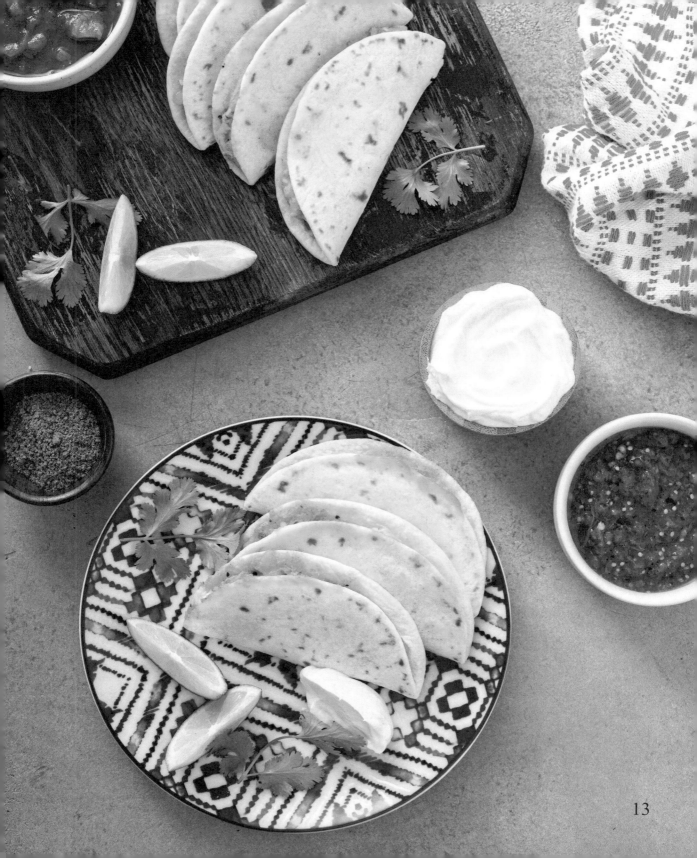

Research and Facts about the Connection Between Nutrition and Alzheimer's Prevention

In recent years, a growing body of scientific research has shed light on the profound influence of nutrition on brain health and the prevention of Alzheimer's disease. Studies have shown that certain dietary patterns and specific nutrients can play a crucial role in reducing the risk of cognitive decline and preserving cognitive function as we age.

The Mediterranean Diet and Cognitive Health

One of the most extensively studied dietary patterns in relation to brain health is the Mediterranean diet. Characterized by high consumption of fruits, vegetables, whole grains, legumes, nuts, seeds, and olive oil, and moderate intake of fish, poultry, and red wine, the Mediterranean diet has been consistently associated with a lower risk of Alzheimer's disease and better cognitive function in older adults.

The DASH Diet and Cognitive Function

Similarly, the DASH (Dietary Approaches to Stop Hypertension) diet, which emphasizes fruits, vegetables, whole grains, lean proteins, and low-fat dairy products while limiting sodium intake, has been linked to a reduced risk of cognitive decline and dementia.

The MIND Diet: A Hybrid Approach

Building on the principles of the Mediterranean and DASH diets, the MIND diet combines the best of both worlds to create a dietary pattern specifically tailored to promote brain health and reduce the risk of Alzheimer's disease. Studies have shown that adherence to the MIND diet is associated with a significant reduction in the risk of Alzheimer's disease, even among individuals who only partially adhere to the diet.

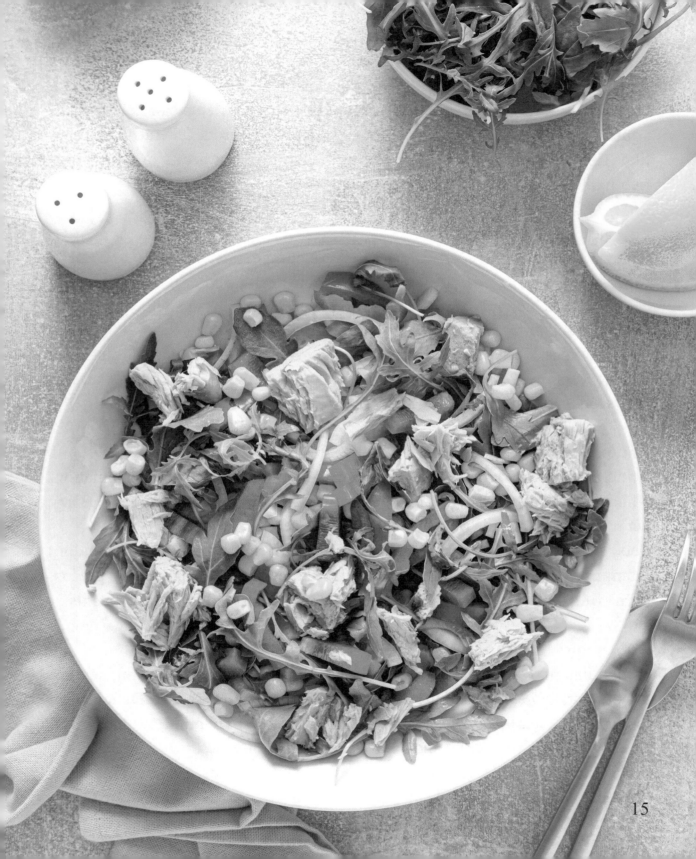

Key Nutrients for Brain Health

Maintaining optimal brain health requires a well-rounded diet rich in key nutrients that support cognitive function, memory, and overall brain health. Incorporating foods that are high in these essential nutrients can help nourish your brain and protect against cognitive decline and neurodegenerative diseases like Alzheimer's. Here are some key nutrients for brain health and the foods rich in them:

Omega-3 Fatty Acids:
Omega-3 fatty acids, particularly EPA (eicosapentaenoic acid) and DHA (docosahexaenoic acid), are crucial for brain health and cognitive function. These fats are integral components of brain cell membranes and play a key role in neurotransmitter signaling.
Food sources: Fatty fish such as salmon, mackerel, trout, and sardines are excellent sources of omega-3 fatty acids. Plant-based sources include flaxseeds, chia seeds, walnuts, and hemp seeds.

Antioxidants:
Antioxidants help protect the brain from oxidative stress and inflammation, which are implicated in neurodegenerative diseases like Alzheimer's. They neutralize harmful free radicals and support overall brain health.
Food sources: Colorful fruits and vegetables are rich in antioxidants, including vitamins C and E, beta-carotene, and flavonoids. Berries, dark leafy greens, citrus fruits, bell peppers, and tomatoes are particularly high in antioxidants.

B Vitamins:
B vitamins play a crucial role in brain health and cognitive function, serving as cofactors in neurotransmitter synthesis and energy metabolism. Deficiencies in certain B vitamins, such as folate, vitamin B6, and vitamin B12, have been linked to cognitive decline and neurodegenerative diseases.
Food sources: Whole grains, leafy greens, legumes, nuts, seeds, eggs, dairy products, poultry, fish, and lean meats are all good sources of B vitamins.

16

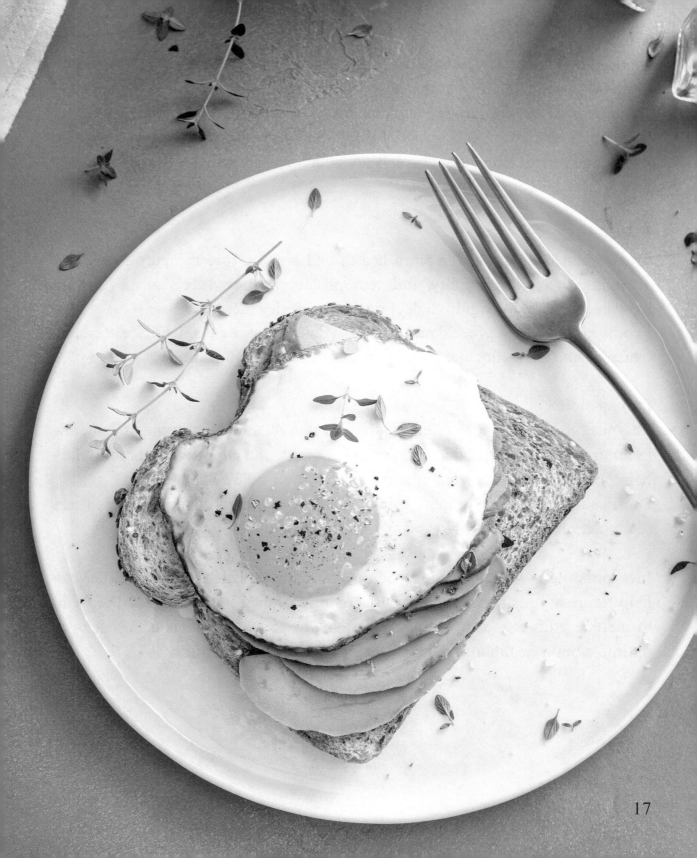

Vitamin D:

Vitamin D is important for brain health and cognitive function, as well as overall immune system function. Low levels of vitamin D have been associated with an increased risk of cognitive decline and Alzheimer's disease.

Food sources: Fatty fish, fortified dairy and plant-based milk alternatives, egg yolks, and fortified breakfast cereals are sources of vitamin D. Sun exposure is also a natural source of vitamin D.

Magnesium:

Magnesium is essential for brain health and plays a role in neurotransmitter signaling, synaptic plasticity, and neuroprotection. Low levels of magnesium have been linked to cognitive decline and neurodegenerative diseases.

Food sources: Leafy greens, nuts, seeds, whole grains, beans, lentils, avocados, bananas, and dark chocolate are good sources of magnesium.

Polyphenols:

Polyphenols are a diverse group of plant compounds with antioxidant and anti-inflammatory properties that support brain health and cognitive function. They help protect brain cells from damage and promote neuroplasticity.

Food sources: Berries, grapes, apples, citrus fruits, dark chocolate, green tea, red wine, olive oil, nuts, seeds, and spices are rich sources of polyphenols.

Incorporating a variety of foods rich in these key nutrients into your diet can help nourish your brain and support cognitive function throughout life. Aim to include a diverse array of nutrient-rich foods in your meals and snacks to optimize brain health and reduce the risk of cognitive decline.

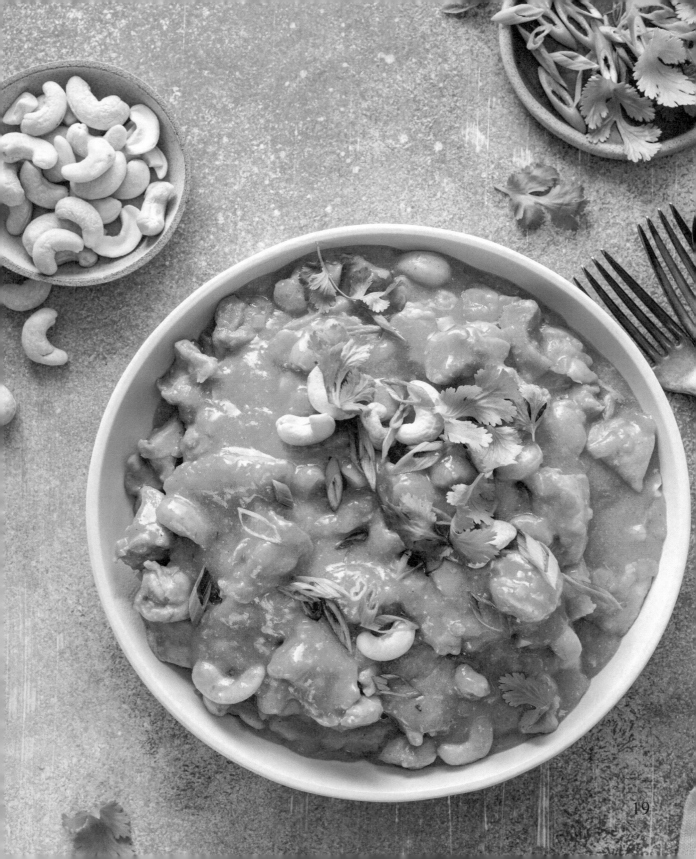

KEY COMPONENTS
OF THE MIND DIET

The MIND diet is characterized by its emphasis on foods that have been shown to promote brain health and cognitive function while discouraging the consumption of those linked to cognitive decline. By following the key components of the MIND diet, individuals can nourish their brains with the nutrients they need to thrive and reduce their risk of developing Alzheimer's disease and other neurodegenerative conditions.

Emphasis on Leafy Greens and Vegetables
Leafy greens, such as spinach, kale, and collard greens, are rich sources of vitamins, minerals, and antioxidants that are essential for brain health. These nutrient-dense foods are associated with slower cognitive decline and a reduced risk of Alzheimer's disease.

Regular Consumption of Berries
Berries, particularly blueberries and strawberries, are powerhouse fruits packed with flavonoids, antioxidants that have been shown to improve cognitive function and protect against age-related cognitive decline. Including a variety of berries in your diet can help support brain health and memory.

Incorporation of Whole Grains
Whole grains, such as oats, quinoa, brown rice, and whole wheat, are rich sources of fiber, vitamins, and minerals that support overall health, including brain health. Consuming whole grains provides a steady supply of energy to the brain and helps maintain stable blood sugar levels, which are essential for cognitive function.

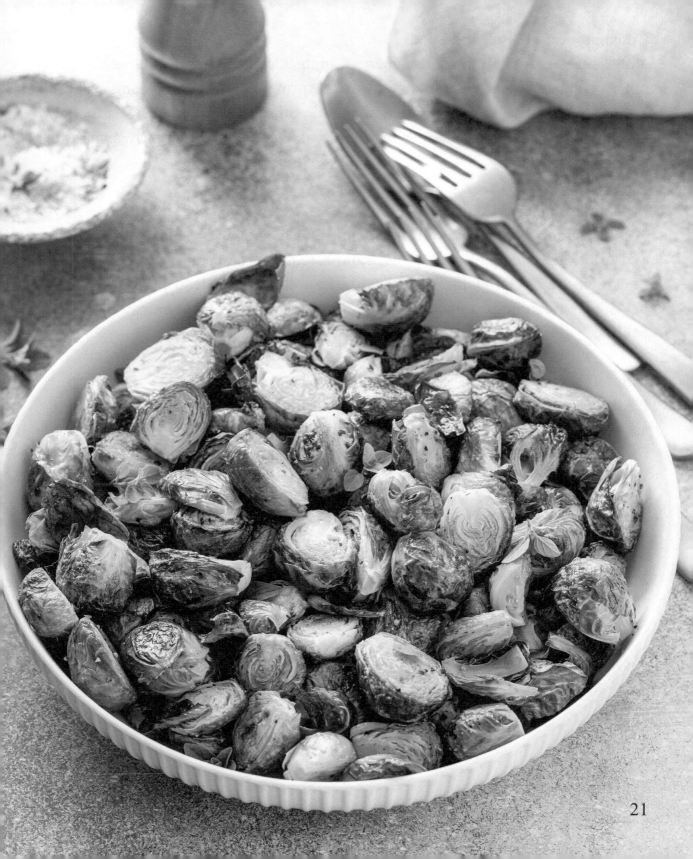

Consumption of Nuts and Seeds

Nuts and seeds, including almonds, walnuts, flaxseeds, and chia seeds, are nutrient-dense foods rich in healthy fats, protein, and antioxidants. These brain-boosting snacks have been associated with improved cognitive function and a reduced risk of Alzheimer's disease when consumed regularly as part of a balanced diet.

Moderate Intake of Poultry and Fish

Poultry, such as chicken and turkey, and fatty fish, such as salmon, mackerel, and trout, are excellent sources of lean protein and omega-3 fatty acids, both of which are essential for brain health. Including these lean protein sources in your diet can help support cognitive function and protect against cognitive decline.

Limited Consumption of Red Meat and Sweets

Red meat and sweets should be consumed sparingly on the MIND diet, as they are associated with an increased risk of cognitive decline and Alzheimer's disease. Instead, focus on incorporating lean protein sources and natural sweeteners, such as fruit, into your diet to support brain health.

Healthy Fats from Olive Oil

Olive oil is a staple of the Mediterranean diet and a key component of the MIND diet. Rich in monounsaturated fats and antioxidants, olive oil has been shown to have numerous health benefits, including protecting against cognitive decline and reducing the risk of Alzheimer's disease.

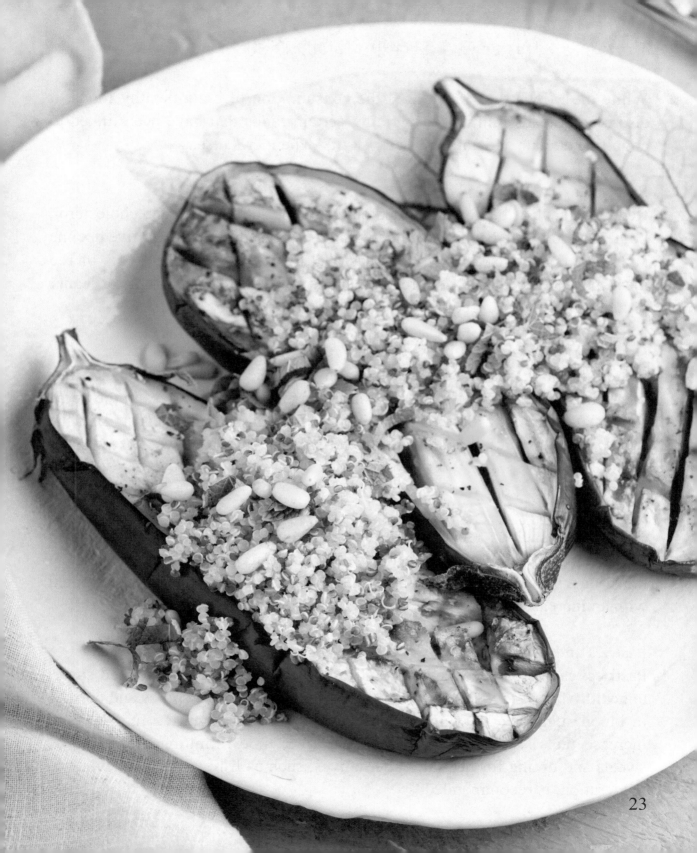

Foods to Limit or Avoid on the MIND Diet

While the MIND diet encourages the consumption of brain-healthy foods, it also recommends limiting or avoiding certain foods that have been linked to cognitive decline and an increased risk of Alzheimer's disease.

Red Meat

Red meat, such as beef, pork, and lamb, is high in saturated fat and cholesterol, both of which have been associated with an increased risk of cognitive decline and Alzheimer's disease. While occasional consumption of lean cuts of red meat may be acceptable, it is recommended to limit intake and opt for leaner protein sources more frequently.

Butter and Margarine

Butter and margarine are high in unhealthy fats, including saturated and trans fats, which have been linked to inflammation and oxidative stress in the body. These fats may contribute to cognitive decline and should be limited on the MIND diet. Instead, choose healthier fat sources such as olive oil, avocado, and nuts.

Fried Foods

Fried foods, such as French fries, fried chicken, and onion rings, are high in unhealthy fats and calories and often contain harmful compounds formed during the frying process. Regular consumption of fried foods has been associated with an increased risk of obesity, heart disease, and cognitive decline.

Pastries and Sweets

Pastries, cakes, cookies, candies, and other sweets are high in refined sugar, unhealthy fats, and empty calories. These foods can lead to spikes and crashes in blood sugar levels, which may negatively impact cognitive function and increase the risk of Alzheimer's disease over time. Limiting the intake of sweets and opting for healthier alternatives, such as fruit or dark chocolate in moderation, is recommended.

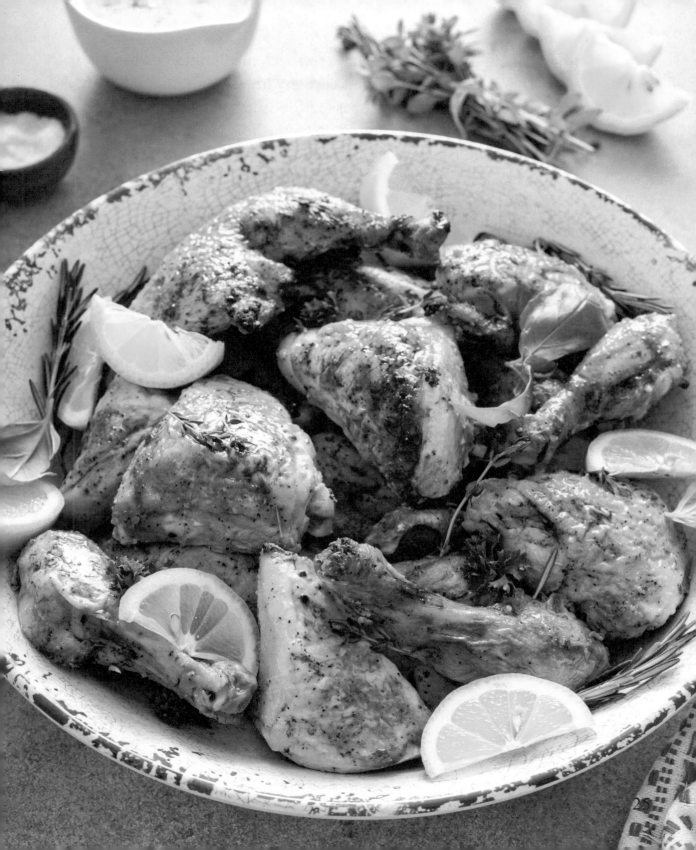

Processed Foods

Processed foods, including packaged snacks, frozen meals, and fast food items, are often high in unhealthy fats, refined carbohydrates, sodium, and artificial additives. Regular consumption of processed foods has been linked to obesity, inflammation, and cognitive decline. Choosing whole, minimally processed foods whenever possible is key to supporting brain health on the MIND diet.

Full-Fat Dairy Products

Full-fat dairy products, such as whole milk, cheese, and cream, are high in saturated fat and cholesterol and should be consumed in moderation on the MIND diet. Opting for low-fat or fat-free dairy options can help reduce saturated fat intake and support heart and brain health.

Sugary Beverages

Sugary beverages, including soda, fruit juices, energy drinks, and sweetened teas, are loaded with added sugars and provide little to no nutritional value. Excessive consumption of sugary beverages has been associated with weight gain, insulin resistance, and cognitive decline. Choosing water, herbal tea, or unsweetened beverages instead can help maintain hydration and support brain health.

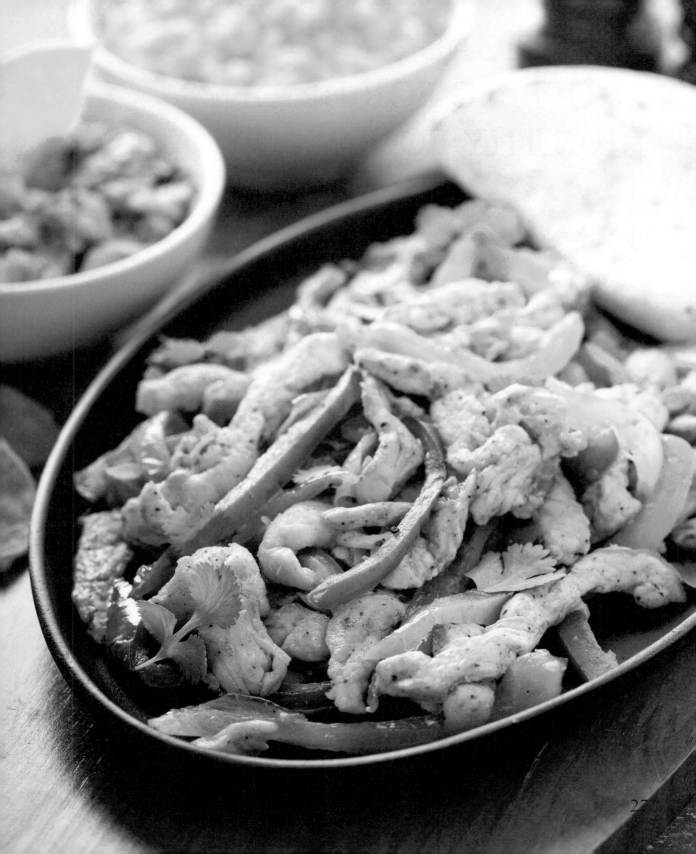

PRACTICAL TIPS FOR SHOPPING FOR BRAIN-HEALTHY FOODS

Navigating the grocery store aisles can sometimes feel overwhelming, especially when trying to make choices that support brain health. However, with a little planning and knowledge, you can shop smart and fill your cart with foods that nourish your brain and support overall well-being. Here are some practical tips to help you shop for brain-healthy foods:

Make a Shopping List

Before heading to the store, take some time to plan your meals for the week and make a shopping list based on the MIND diet principles. Include a variety of fruits, vegetables, whole grains, lean proteins, nuts, seeds, and healthy fats on your list, and try to choose foods from each category to ensure a balanced diet.

Shop the Perimeter

When you arrive at the grocery store, start by shopping the perimeter, where you'll find fresh produce, meats, dairy, and other whole foods. Focus on filling your cart with colorful fruits and vegetables, lean proteins like poultry and fish, and whole grains like brown rice, quinoa, and oats. These foods are rich in nutrients that support brain health and overall well-being.

Read Labels

As you shop, take the time to read labels and ingredients lists to make informed choices about the foods you buy. Look for products that are low in added sugars, unhealthy fats, and artificial additives, and choose whole, minimally processed foods whenever possible. Pay attention to serving sizes and nutrient content to ensure you're getting the most nutritional bang for your buck.

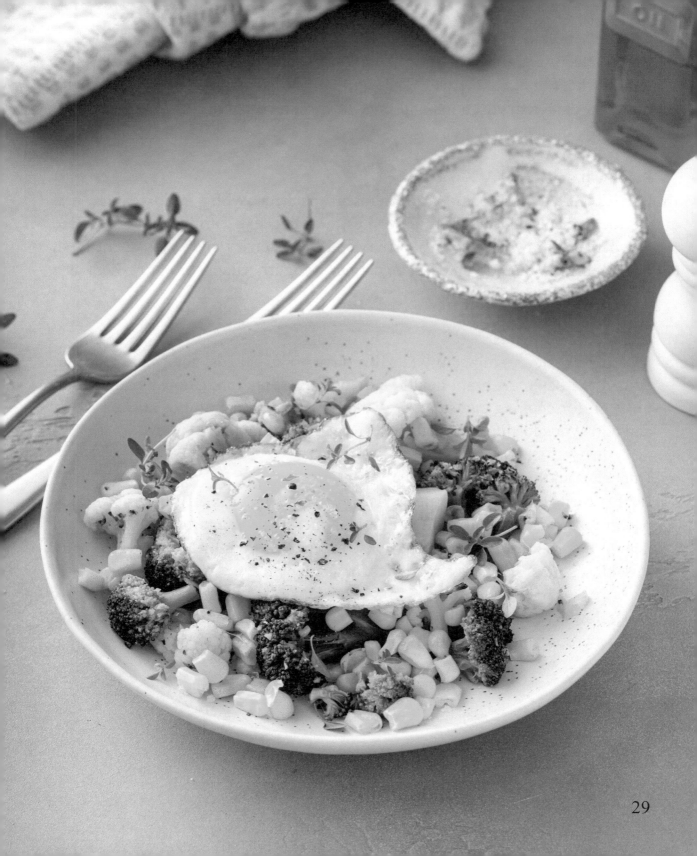

Choose Whole Grains

When selecting grains, opt for whole grains like brown rice, quinoa, barley, and whole wheat bread and pasta. These grains are higher in fiber, vitamins, and minerals than refined grains and provide sustained energy to fuel your brain and body throughout the day.

Stock Up on Berries

Berries are nutritional powerhouses packed with antioxidants and phytochemicals that support brain health. Choose a variety of berries like blueberries, strawberries, raspberries, and blackberries and enjoy them fresh or frozen. Add them to smoothies, oatmeal, yogurt, salads, or enjoy them as a healthy snack on their own.

Include Healthy Fats

Incorporate sources of healthy fats like olive oil, avocados, nuts, and seeds into your diet to support brain health and cognitive function. Choose extra-virgin olive oil for cooking and salad dressings, snack on a handful of nuts or seeds, and add avocado slices to sandwiches, salads, or wraps.

Don't Forget the Leafy Greens

Leafy greens like spinach, kale, collard greens, and Swiss chard are nutritional powerhouses rich in vitamins, minerals, and antioxidants that support brain health. Incorporate these nutrient-dense greens into your meals by adding them to salads, soups, stir-fries, smoothies, or sandwiches.

By following these practical tips, you can make shopping for brain-healthy foods a breeze and set yourself up for success on the MIND diet.

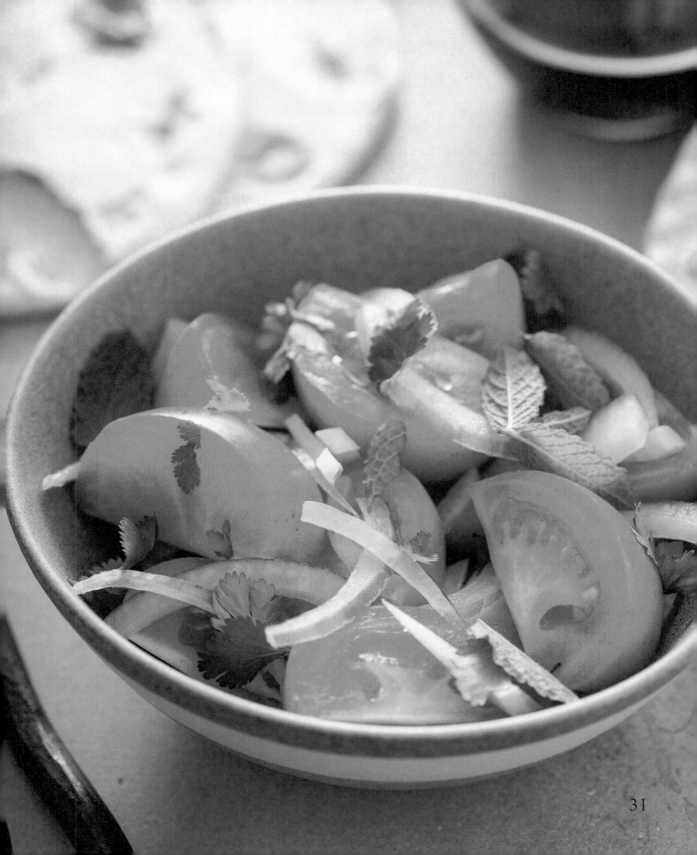

Reading Labels: Identifying Nutrients Beneficial for Brain Health

Understanding how to read food labels can empower you to make informed choices that support brain health. By paying attention to key nutrients and ingredients, you can select foods that provide the vitamins, minerals, and antioxidants your brain needs to function optimally. Here are some tips for reading labels and identifying nutrients beneficial for brain health:

Look for High Fiber Content

Fiber is important for maintaining stable blood sugar levels and supporting digestive health, which in turn can impact brain function. Choose foods that are high in fiber, such as whole grains, fruits, vegetables, nuts, and seeds. Look for products that contain at least 3 grams of fiber per serving, and opt for whole grain varieties whenever possible.

Check the Sugar Content

High sugar intake has been linked to cognitive decline and an increased risk of Alzheimer's disease. Limit your consumption of added sugars by choosing products with minimal added sugars and opting for naturally sweetened options like fruit. Be wary of hidden sugars in processed foods, and avoid products with ingredients like corn syrup, cane sugar, and high fructose corn syrup.

Assess the Fat Profile

Healthy fats, such as monounsaturated and polyunsaturated fats, are essential for brain health and cognitive function. Look for products that contain healthy fats from sources like olive oil, avocados, nuts, and seeds. Avoid products that are high in saturated and trans fats, which have been linked to cognitive decline and heart disease.

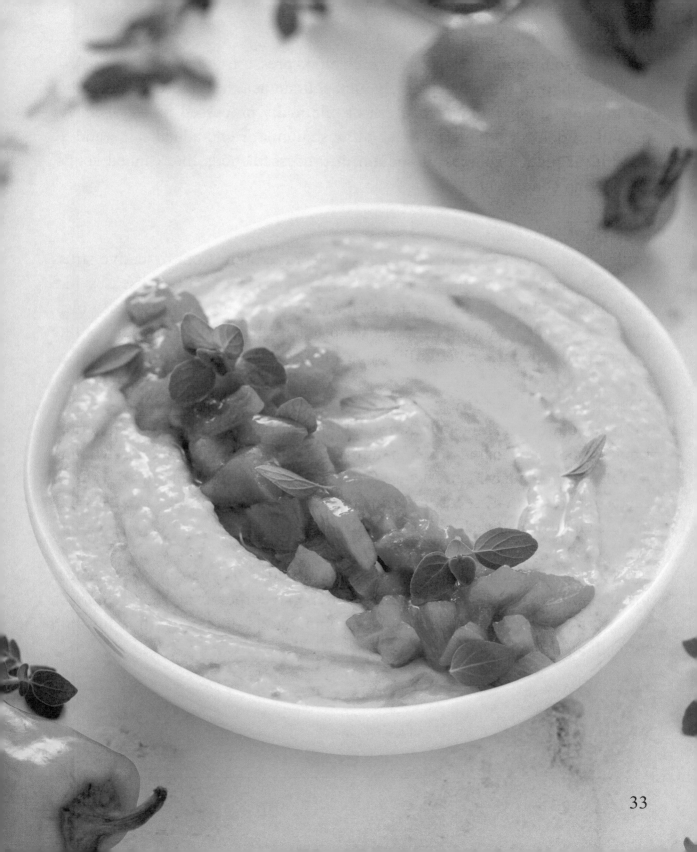

Check the Sodium Content

Excessive sodium intake can lead to high blood pressure and increase the risk of stroke, both of which can negatively impact brain health. Choose products that are low in sodium, and opt for fresh or minimally processed foods whenever possible. Look for products labeled «low sodium» or «no added salt,» and be mindful of hidden sources of sodium in processed foods like canned soups, sauces, and condiments.

Seek Out Antioxidants

Antioxidants are compounds that help protect the brain from oxidative stress and inflammation, which are implicated in neurodegenerative diseases like Alzheimer's. Choose foods that are rich in antioxidants, such as fruits, vegetables, nuts, seeds, and whole grains. Look for products that contain ingredients like berries, leafy greens, and colorful fruits and vegetables.

Check for Essential Nutrients

Certain vitamins and minerals are crucial for brain health and cognitive function. Look for products that are high in nutrients like vitamin E, vitamin C, vitamin K, folate, and omega-3 fatty acids. These nutrients can be found in a variety of foods, including nuts, seeds, leafy greens, fatty fish, and fortified products like cereals and dairy alternatives.

By reading labels and paying attention to key nutrients, you can make choices that support brain health and overall well-being. Incorporate nutrient-rich foods into your diet regularly to nourish your brain and promote cognitive function throughout life.

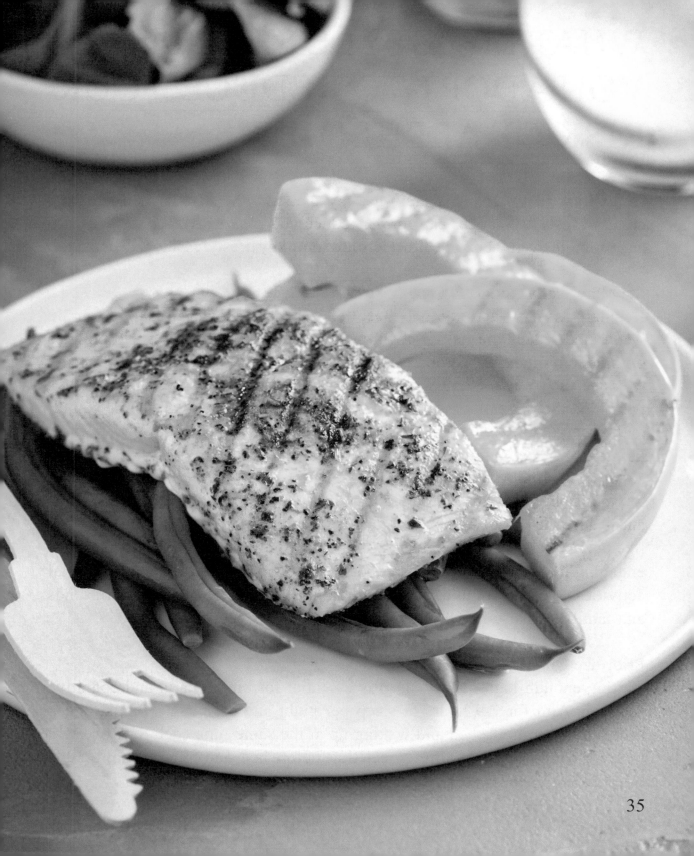

35

WHAT LIFESTYLE SHOULD YOU ADOPT TO REDUCE YOUR RISK OF ALZHEIMER'S

In addition to following a brain-healthy diet like the MIND diet, adopting certain lifestyle practices can further reduce your risk of Alzheimer's disease and promote overall brain health. Here are some key lifestyle factors to consider:

Stay Physically Active
Regular physical activity has been consistently shown to support brain health and reduce the risk of cognitive decline. Aim for at least 150 minutes of moderate-intensity aerobic exercise or 75 minutes of vigorous-intensity exercise each week, along with strength training exercises two or more days per week. Activities like walking, swimming, dancing, and gardening can all help keep your brain sharp and your body healthy.

Keep Your Mind Active
Engaging in mentally stimulating activities can help build cognitive reserve and reduce the risk of Alzheimer's disease. Challenge your brain with activities like puzzles, crosswords, sudoku, reading, learning a new skill or language, or engaging in hobbies that require problem-solving and critical thinking. Social activities, such as volunteering, joining clubs, or spending time with friends and family, can also help keep your brain sharp and your mood lifted.

Prioritize Quality Sleep
Getting enough high-quality sleep is essential for brain health and cognitive function. Aim for 7-9 hours of sleep per night and establish a regular sleep schedule by going to bed and waking up at the same time each day. Create a relaxing bedtime routine, limit screen time before bed, and create a comfortable sleep environment free of distractions to promote restful sleep.

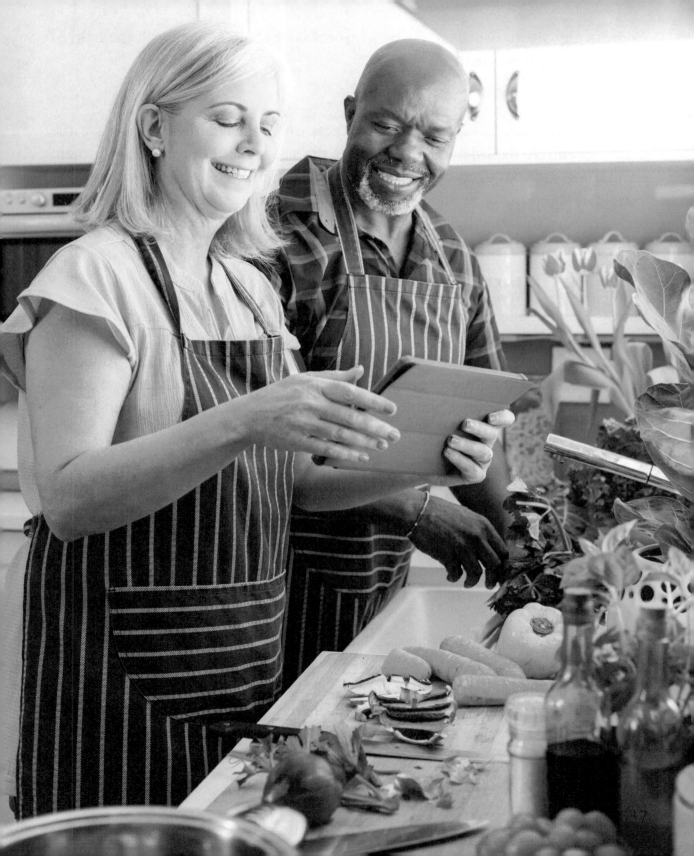

Address any sleep disorders, such as insomnia or sleep apnea, with the help of a healthcare professional.

Manage Stress

Chronic stress can have detrimental effects on brain health and increase the risk of cognitive decline and Alzheimer's disease. Practice stress management techniques such as deep breathing, meditation, yoga, tai chi, or progressive muscle relaxation to promote relaxation and reduce stress levels. Prioritize self-care activities that help you unwind and recharge, such as spending time in nature, practicing mindfulness, or pursuing hobbies you enjoy.

Maintain Social Connections

Strong social connections are vital for brain health and overall well-being. Stay connected with friends, family, and community members through regular social activities, phone calls, video chats, or in-person gatherings. Join clubs, volunteer organizations, or community groups to meet new people and stay engaged with others. Social interaction stimulates the brain, promotes emotional well-being, and reduces the risk of cognitive decline.

Protect Your Brain

Take steps to protect your brain from injury and harm. Wear a helmet when engaging in activities like biking, skiing, or skating, and use seat belts and other safety equipment when driving or participating in sports. Avoid activities that pose a risk of head injury, such as contact sports or risky behaviors like excessive alcohol consumption or substance abuse.

Well, all the secrets are revealed. And I think each of you understands that everything is quite simple. Make your life better, follow these great tips, switch to the MIND diet and you will feel better. I will repeat to you once again my favorite phrase «It is never too early to change your life and develop good habits that may later save your life and allow you to live your older years in peace».

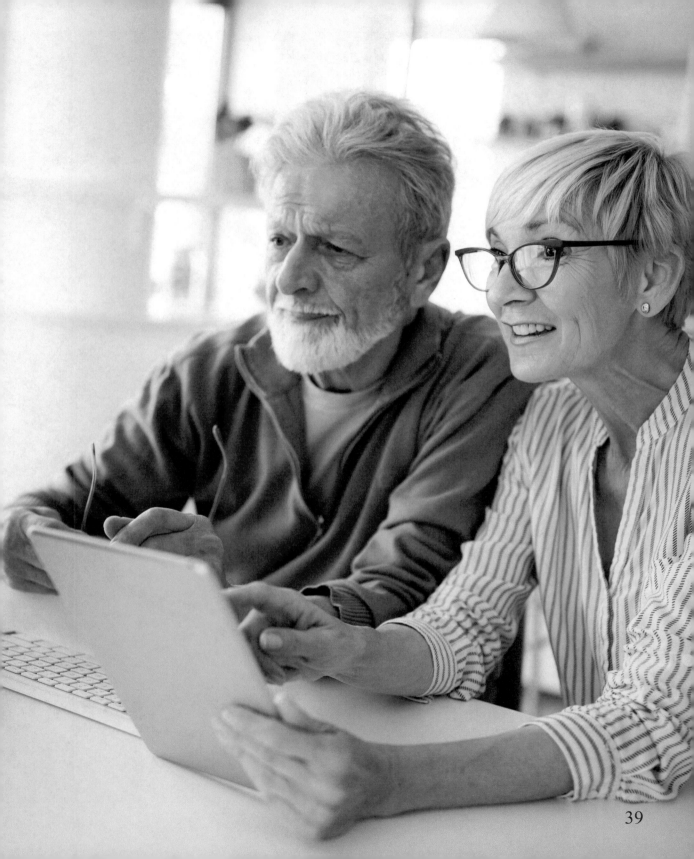

39

BREAKFAST RECIPES

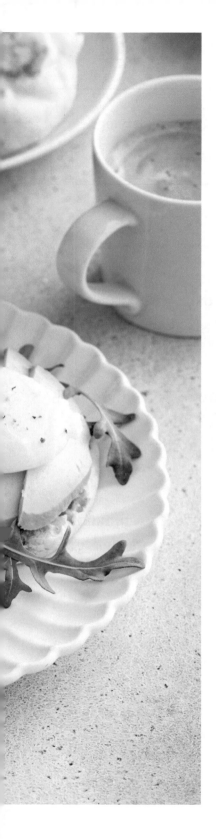

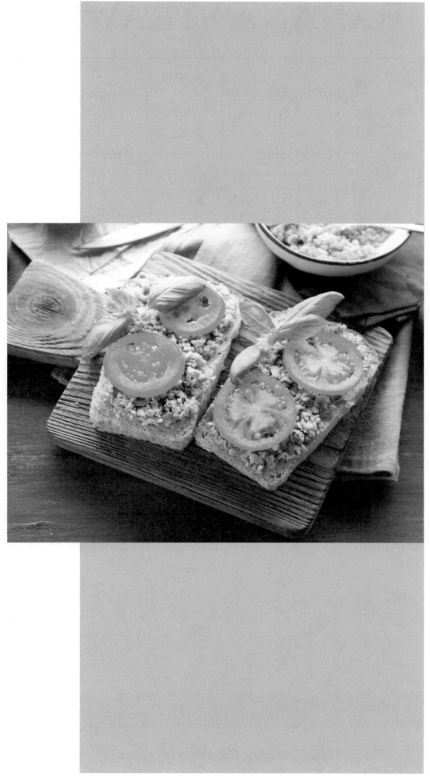

BANANA STRAWBERRY OATS

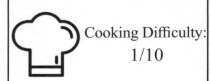 Cooking Difficulty: 1/10

 Cooking Time: 15 minutes

 Servings: 1

INGREDIENTS

- 1 tbsp. sliced almonds
- ½ c. oats
- ½ tsp. cinnamon
- 1 c. shredded zucchini
- ½ banana, mashed
- 1 c. water
- ½ c. sliced strawberries
- dash of salt
- 1 tbsp. flax meal

DESCRIPTION

STEP 1
First, combine oats, salt, water, and zucchini in a large saucepan.

STEP 2
Cook the mixture over medium-high heat and cook for 8 to 10 minutes or until the liquid is absorbed.

STEP 3
Now, spoon in all the remaining ingredients to the mixture and give everything a good stir.

STEP 4
Finally, transfer the mixture to a serving bowl and top it with almonds and strawberries. Serve and enjoy.

NUTRITIONAL INFORMATION

Calories: 386, Proteins: 23.7g, Carbs: 57.5g, Fat: 8.9g

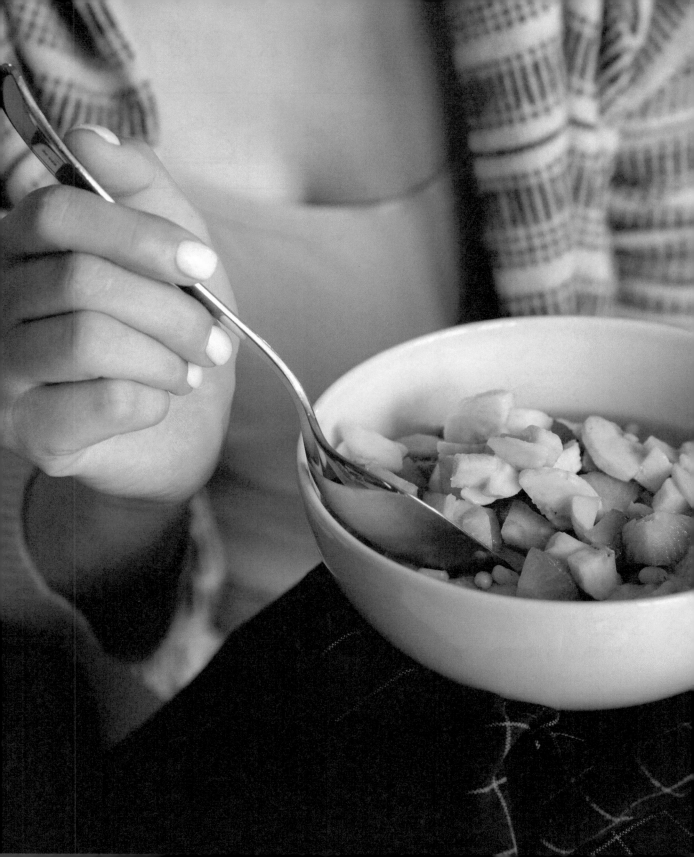

GRANOLA WITH GRAPEFRUIT

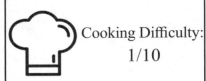 Cooking Difficulty: 1/10

 Cooking Time: 3 minutes

 Servings: 2

INGREDIENTS

- 1/2 cup coconut cream
- 6 tbsp. granola
- grapefruit

DESCRIPTION

STEP 1
Take two cups. Place 3 spoonfuls of granola in each one.

STEP 2
Then place the coconut cream on top of the granola.

STEP 3
Garnish everything with grapefruit. Enjoy your meal.

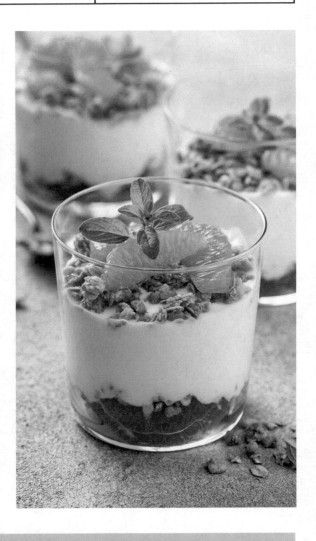

NUTRITIONAL INFORMATION

111 Calories, 6g Fats, 3g Carbs, 6.8 Protein

CHIA SEED PUDDING

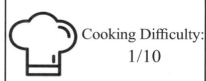 Cooking Difficulty: 1/10

 Cooking Time: 12 minutes

 Servings: 1

INGREDIENTS

- 1/2 cup coconut milk
- 2 tbsp. chia seeds
- berries

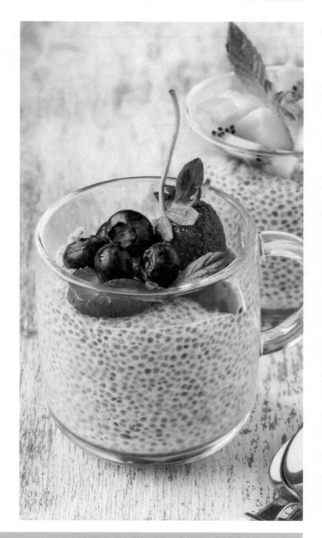

DESCRIPTION

STEP 1

Combine chia seeds and milk in a large bowl. Let the mixture sit for 10 minutes, then stir again as soon as the chia seeds begin to swell.

STEP 2

Cover the bowl with a lid and refrigerate for an hour or more. Stir the chia pudding before serving and add your favorite berries. Enjoy!

NUTRITIONAL INFORMATION

180 Calories, 3 g Fat, 3g Carbs, 3g Protein

CHIA CINNAMON VANILLA GRANOLA

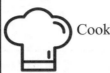 Cooking Difficulty: 3/10

 Cooking Time: 29 minutes

 Servings: 6

INGREDIENTS

- 56g whey protein powder
- 1 c. macadamia nuts
- ¼ c. water
- 4 tbsps. flaxseed meal
- 4 tbsps. whole chia seeds
- 4 tbsps. coconut oil, melted
- 3 tbsps. water
- 4 tsps. stevia
- 2 tsps. cinnamon
- 1 tsp. pure vanilla extract
- ¼ tsp. fine sea salt

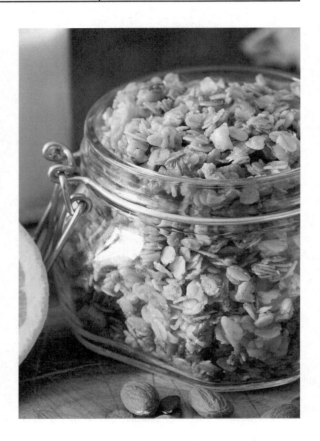

NUTRITIONAL INFORMATION

336 Calories, 21g Fats, 11g Carbs, and 9g Protein

DESCRIPTION

STEP 1
Set the oven to 350 degrees F to preheat. Line a baking sheet with baking paper and set it aside.

STEP 2
Mix together the vanilla extract, water, and chia seeds in a large bowl. Set aside for 5 minutes, or until the mixture becomes gelatinous.

STEP 3
Pour the macadamia nuts into a food processor, then add the flaxseed meal, protein powder, stevia, salt, and cinnamon. Pulse until the mixture is fine and the nuts are grounded.

STEP 4
Pour the gelatinous chia seed mixture into the food processor, then add about 1 ½ tablespoon of water and the coconut oil. Blend until the mixture is smooth. Set aside.

STEP 5
Using a tablespoon, transfer the mixture onto the prepared baking sheet. Then, transfer to the oven and bake for 15 minutes.

STEP 6
Once baked, remove from the oven and break into small pieces. Spread out on the pan.

STEP 7
Bake for an additional 10 minutes, or until the granola is dry and golden brown. Set on a cooling rack and allow to cool completely. Transfer to an airtight container and store for up to 1 week in the refrigerator. Best served with warm milk.

TOMATOES AND EGGS

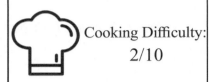 Cooking Difficulty: 2/10

 Cooking Time: 15 minutes

 Servings: 2

INGREDIENTS

- 1 tbsp. olive oil
- salt
- black pepper
- dried basil
- 1 tbsp. chopped parsley
- 4 eggs
- 6 tomatoes diced

DESCRIPTION

STEP 1
Heat olive oil in a pan.

STEP 2
Add tomatoes, spices, and herbs. Simmer, stirring, for about 5-7 minutes.

STEP 3
Make small wells in the sauce and break the eggs into them. Season with salt and cook until the white is white and the yolk inside is still runny.

STEP 4
Remove from fire. Sprinkle with parsley before serving.

NUTRITIONAL INFORMATION

Calories: 710, Fat: 4 g, Carbs: 5 g, Protein: 3 g

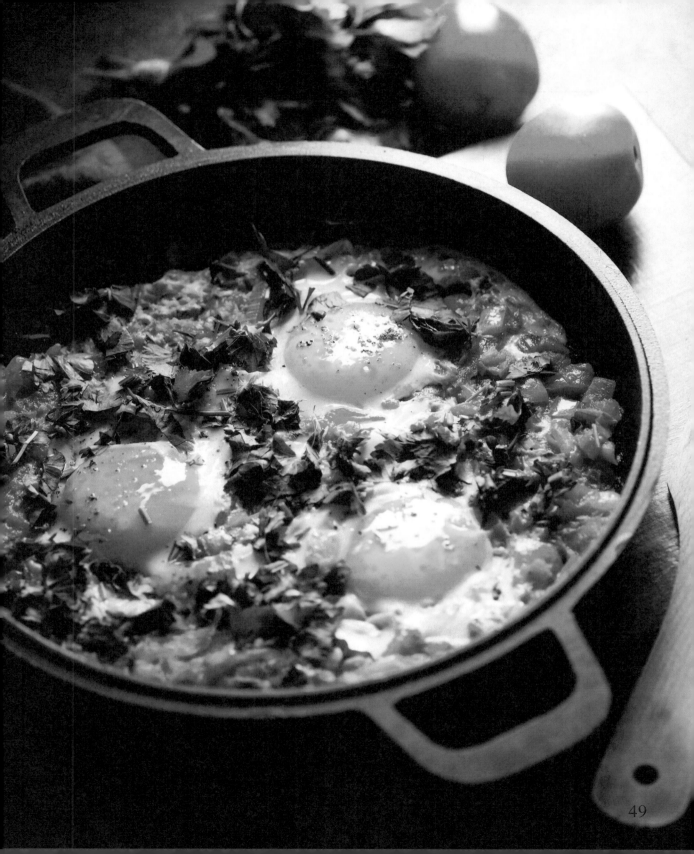

TOFU SCRAMBLE TOAST

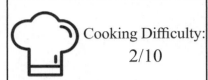 Cooking Difficulty: 2/10

 Cooking Time: 7 minutes

 Servings: 2

INGREDIENTS

- 14 ounces of drained and diced tofu
- ½ yellow onion
- 2 teaspoons cajun seasoning
- 2 toasted bread
- favorite vegetables for serving

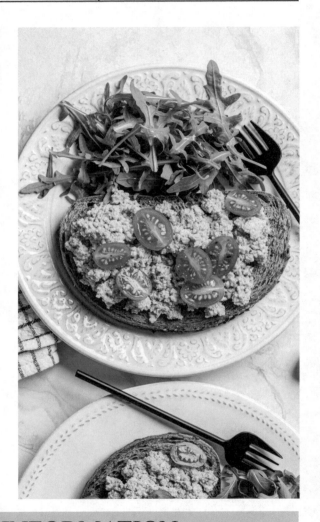

DESCRIPTION

STEP 1

Heat a frying pan and add a little olive oil. Add tofu and spices. Cook for 5 minutes. Fry one side of the toast. Place tofu on toast. Garnish with your favorite vegetables. Serve for breakfast.

NUTRITIONAL INFORMATION

247 Calories, 5.8g Fats, 6g Carbs, 10g Protein

SALMON TOAST

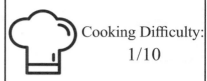 **Cooking Difficulty:** 1/10

 Cooking Time: 3 minutes

 Servings: 2

INGREDIENTS

- lightly salted salmon
- 1 cucumber
- vegan cream cheese
- 4 toasted bread slices

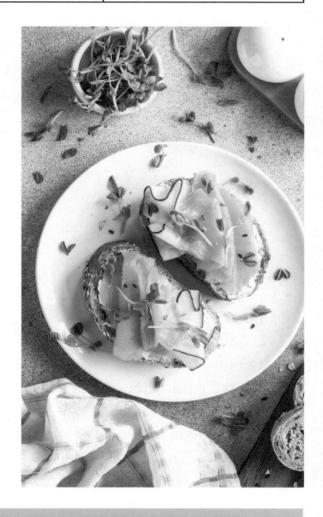

DESCRIPTION

STEP 1
Slice the cucumber into slices.

STEP 2
Spread cream cheese on toasted bread. Place lightly salted salmon on top. Garnish with microgreen, if desired. Enjoy your meal.

NUTRITIONAL INFORMATION

Calories: 210, Fat: 4.4 g, Carbs: 3.8 g, Protein: 6 g

BEET HUMMUS TOAST

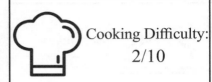 Cooking Difficulty: 2/10

 Cooking Time: 5 minutes

 Servings: 2

INGREDIENTS

- 2 slices of whole-grain bread (preferably rye or oats)
- 1/2 cup beet hummus (recipe below)
- 2 eggs
- salt and pepper to taste
- fresh herbs for garnish (parsley, dill, basil)

beet hummus:
- 1 medium-sized beet, boiled and diced
- 1/2 cup smooth chickpea hummus
- 1 clove garlic, finely chopped
- juice of half a lemon
- 2 tablespoons olive oil

DESCRIPTION

STEP 1
In a blender, combine the boiled beet, chickpea hummus, finely chopped garlic, lemon juice, and olive oil. Blend all the ingredients until you achieve a smooth consistency. Add salt and pepper to taste.

STEP 2
Heat a skillet over medium heat and add a bit of olive oil. Add eggs to a preheated pan and cook until cooked. Season with salt and pepper.

STEP 3
Spread of beet hummus on each slice of toasted bread. Place the cooked eggs on top of the beet hummus. Garnish with fresh herbs.

NUTRITIONAL INFORMATION

283.6 Calories, 11.5g Fat, 31g Carbs, 10.9g Protein

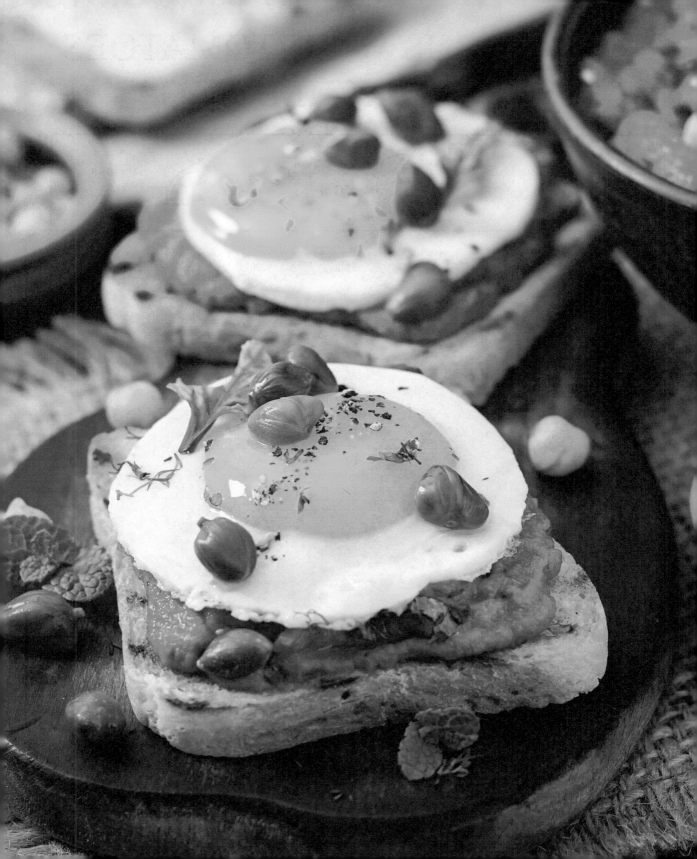

ASPARAGUS WITH TOMATOES AND POACHED EGG

 Cooking Difficulty: 3/10

 Cooking Time: 10 minutes

 Servings: 1

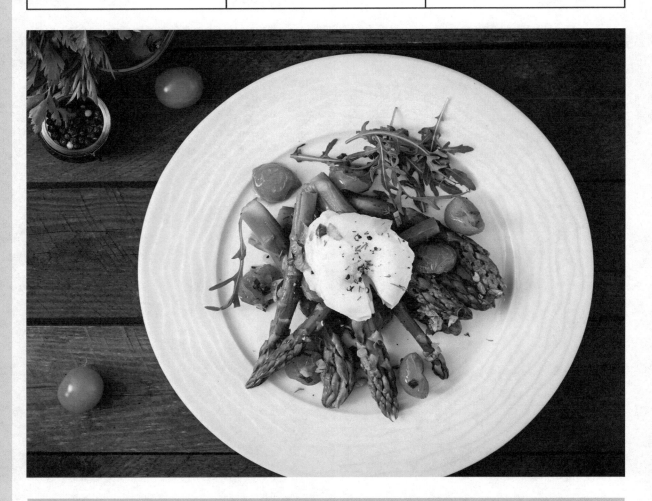

NUTRITIONAL INFORMATION

199 Calories, 7g Fats, 6g Carbs, 6g Protein

INGREDIENTS

- 100g fresh asparagus
- 6-8 cherry tomatoes, halved
- 1 egg
- 1 tablespoon olive oil
- salt and pepper to taste
- fresh herbs for garnish (parsley, basil)

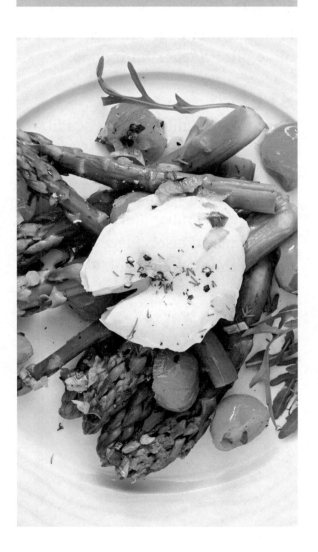

DESCRIPTION

STEP 1

Trim the ends of the asparagus and cut them to your desired length. Heat a skillet with olive oil over medium heat. Sauté the asparagus for 3-5 minutes, adding cherry tomatoes. Sauté until the asparagus is tender, and the tomatoes begin to soften. Season with salt and pepper to taste.

STEP 2

Bring water to a simmer in a shallow saucepan until small bubbles form. Create a vortex in the water by stirring it with a whisk. Carefully crack the egg into the vortex and poach for 3-4 minutes for a soft poached egg.

STEP 3

Arrange the sautéed asparagus with tomatoes on a plate. Place the poached egg on top. Season with salt and pepper to taste. Garnish with fresh herbs. Serve the dish hot and enjoy a delicious and nutritious breakfast!

BREAKFAST CROISSANT

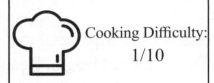 Cooking Difficulty: 1/10

 Cooking Time: 5 minutes

 Servings: 2

INGREDIENTS

- 2 croissants
- 1 cucumber
- 1 avocado
- 2 eggs
- salt, pepper
- arugula (optional)

DESCRIPTION

STEP 1
Heat a skillet over low heat and add olive oil. Fry eggs until done.

STEP 2
Slice the cucumber and avocado.

STEP 3
Slice the croissant. Arrange the arugula, cucumber and avocado. Salt and pepper to taste. Place a fried egg on top. Enjoy your meal.

NUTRITIONAL INFORMATION

Calories: 230, Fat: 4.4 g, Carbs: 5 g, Protein: 5 g

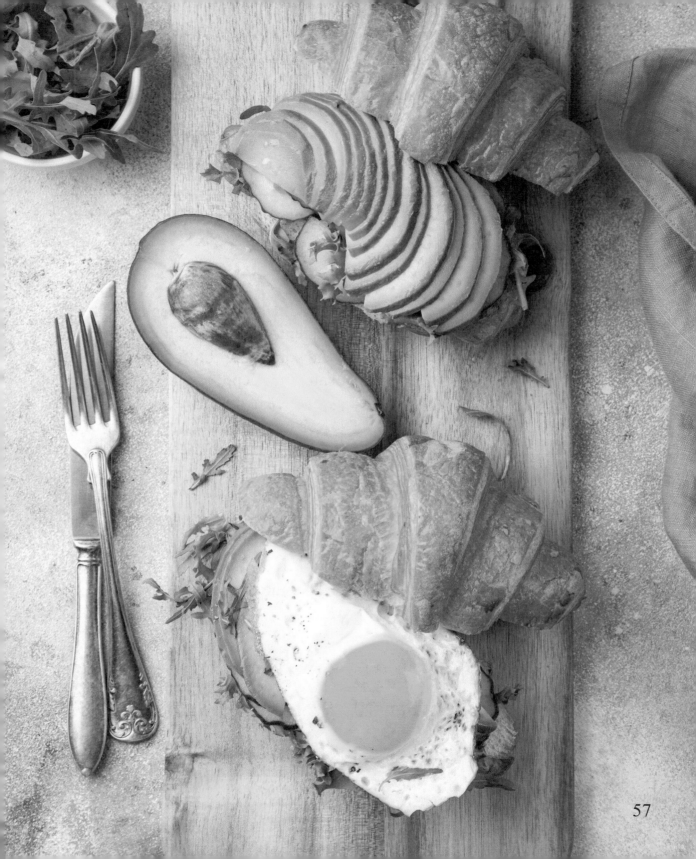

VEGETABLE OMELETTE

 Cooking Difficulty: 2/10

 Cooking Time: 15 minutes

 Servings: 2

INGREDIENTS

- 4 eggs
- 1/4 cup diced tomatoes
- 1/4 cup diced red bell pepper
- 1/4 cup chopped spinach
- Salt and pepper to taste
- 1 teaspoon olive oil

DESCRIPTION

STEP 1
In a bowl, whisk the eggs until well beaten. Add the tomatoes, bell pepper, and spinach to the eggs. Season with salt and pepper to taste, and mix well. Heat the olive oil in a skillet over medium heat. Pour half of the egg mixture into the skillet and cook the omelette, stirring occasionally, until it becomes firm. Repeat with the remaining egg mixture.

STEP 2
Serve the cooked vegetable omelette hot.

NUTRITIONAL INFORMATION

15g Carbs, 10g Fat, 10g Protein, 260 Calories

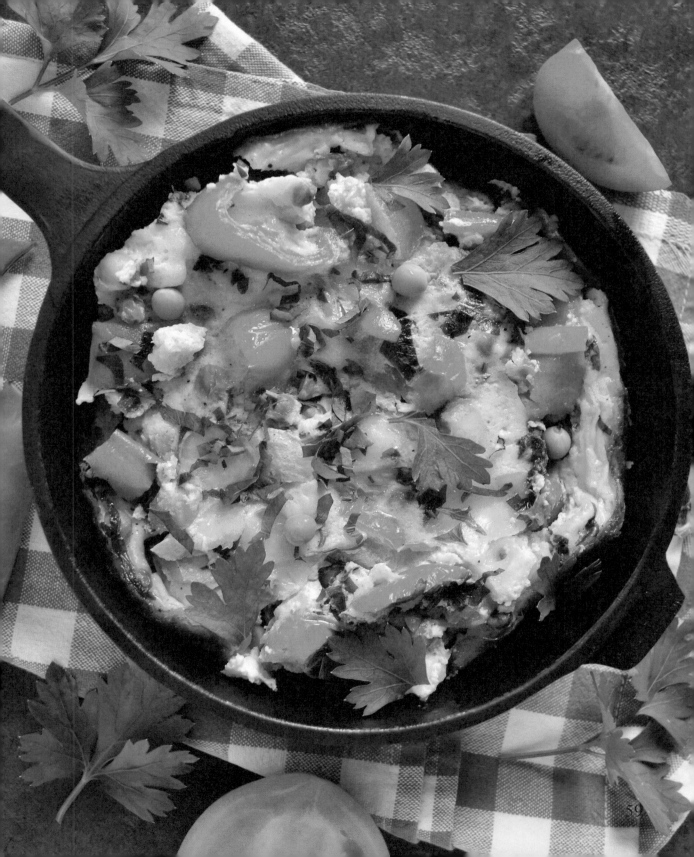

CHOCOLATE QUINOA SOUP

Cooking Difficulty: 2/10	Cooking Time: 22 minutes	Servings: 2

INGREDIENTS

- 1 c. brown quinoa
- 4 c. water
- 2 tbsps. dutch cocoa powder
- ¼ c. chopped dark chocolate (optional)
- 1 c. vegan milk

DESCRIPTION

STEP 1
Pour brown quinoa, water, cocoa powder and dark chocolate into the Instant Pot. Stir mixture well.

STEP 2
Close the lid. Lock in place and make sure to seal the valve. Press the pressure button and cook for 8 minutes on high.

STEP 3
When the timer beeps, choose the quick pressure release. This would take 1–2 minutes. Remove the lid. Adjust taste if needed.

STEP 4
To serve, ladle equal portions into 2 bowls. Pour vegan milk.

NUTRITIONAL INFORMATION

Calories: 116; Fat: 4.3 g; Carbs: 14.1 g; Protein: 3.1 g

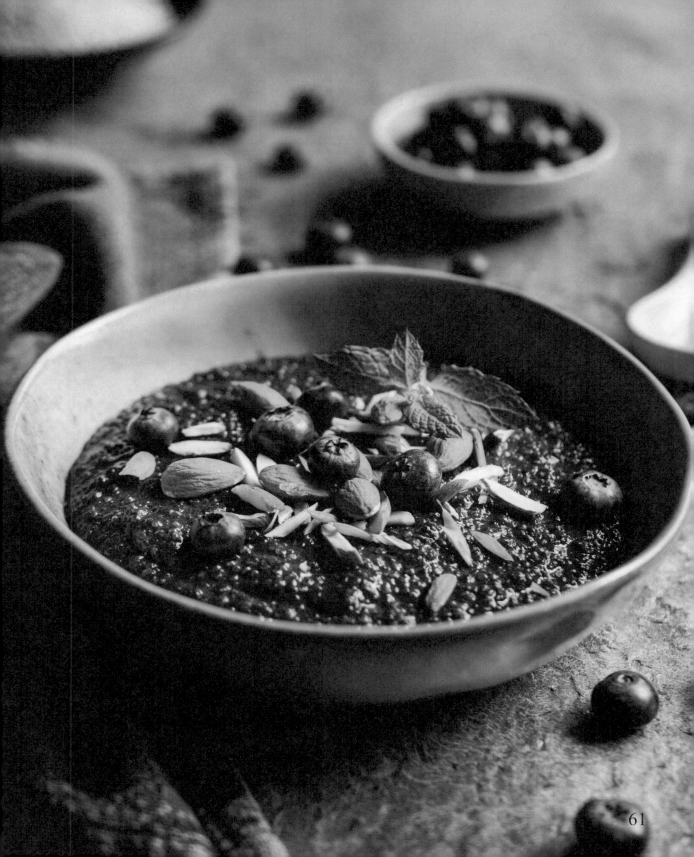

AVOCADO & EGG BREAKFAST SANDWICH

 Cooking Difficulty: 2/10

 Cooking Time: 5 minutes

 Servings: 2

INGREDIENTS

- 4 toasted bread slices
- 1 avocado
- 12 steamed asparagus spears
- 1 sliced hard-boiled egg
- 1 tomato (optional)
- olive oil
- pepper
- sea salt
- dijon mustard

DESCRIPTION

STEP 1
Peel and mash the avocado and toast the bread.

STEP 2
Prepare the sandwich by using the mustard with a layer of avocado.

STEP 3
Add the asparagus spears and eggs. Give it a drizzle of oil along with some salt and pepper. Close and enjoy.

NUTRITIONAL INFORMATION

283.6 Calories, 11.5g Fat, 31g Carbs, 10.9g Protein

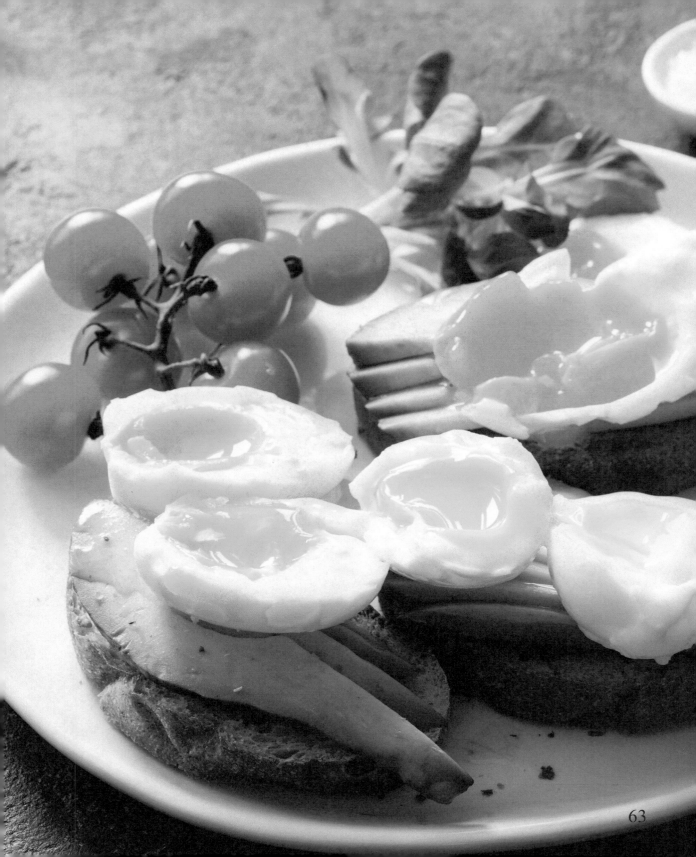

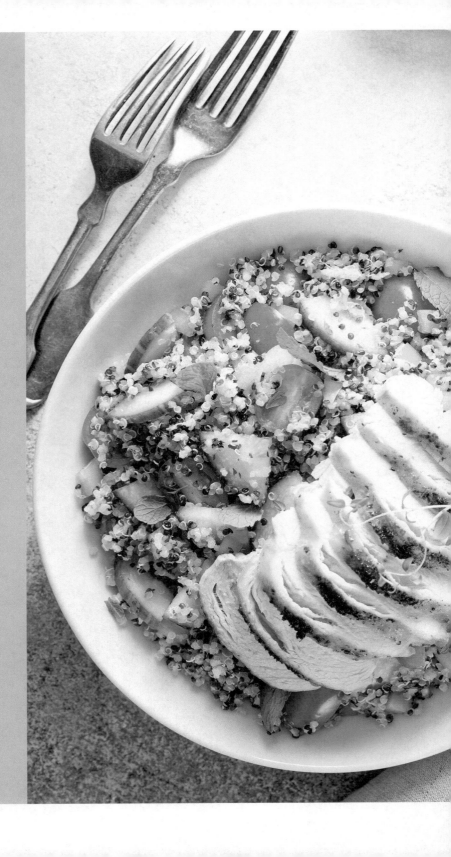

MAIN DISH

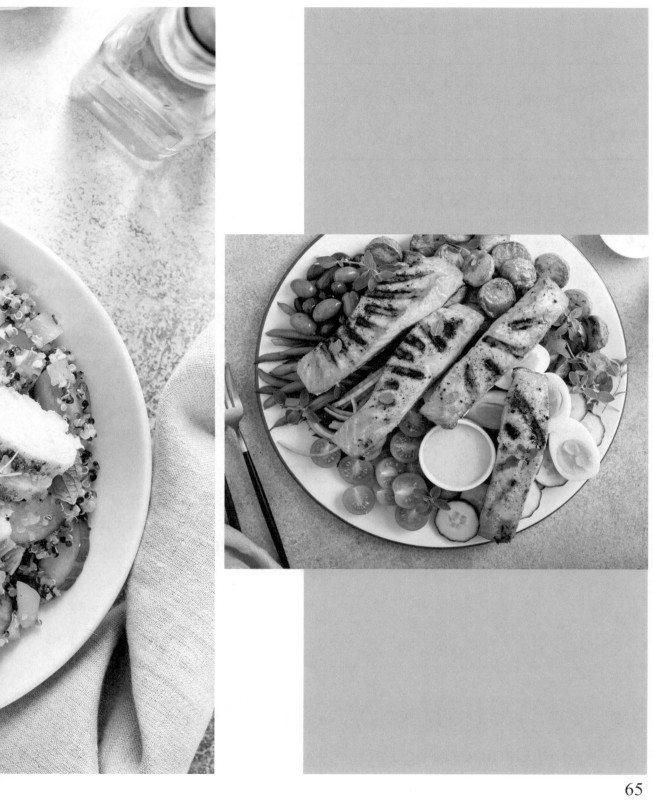

SEA BASS

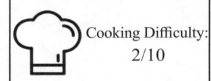 Cooking Difficulty: 2/10

 Cooking Time: 22 minutes

 Servings: 2

INGREDIENTS

- 2 sea bass fillets
- 2 tbsp olive oil
- salt and black pepper to taste
- 1 tsp dried thyme
- 1 tsp mediterranean herb blend (rosemary, basil, oregano)
- 2 cloves garlic, minced
- lemon wedges (for serving)
- fresh herbs (parsley, dill) for garnish

DESCRIPTION

STEP 1
Preheat oven to 400°F (200°C). Make an X-shaped cut into the skin of each sea bass fillet to allow the spices to penetrate. In a bowl, combine olive oil, salt, black pepper, and all remaining spices. Coat the fillets evenly with the marinade, making sure to get it into the cuts in the skin.

STEP 2
Place the fillets on a baking sheet or in a baking dish. Bake in the preheated oven for 15-20 minutes or until the fish easily flakes with a fork.

STEP 3
Serve the baked sea bass hot and pair it with your favorite fresh salad.

NUTRITIONAL INFORMATION

380 Calories, 26g Fats, 3.4g Carbs, 11g Protein

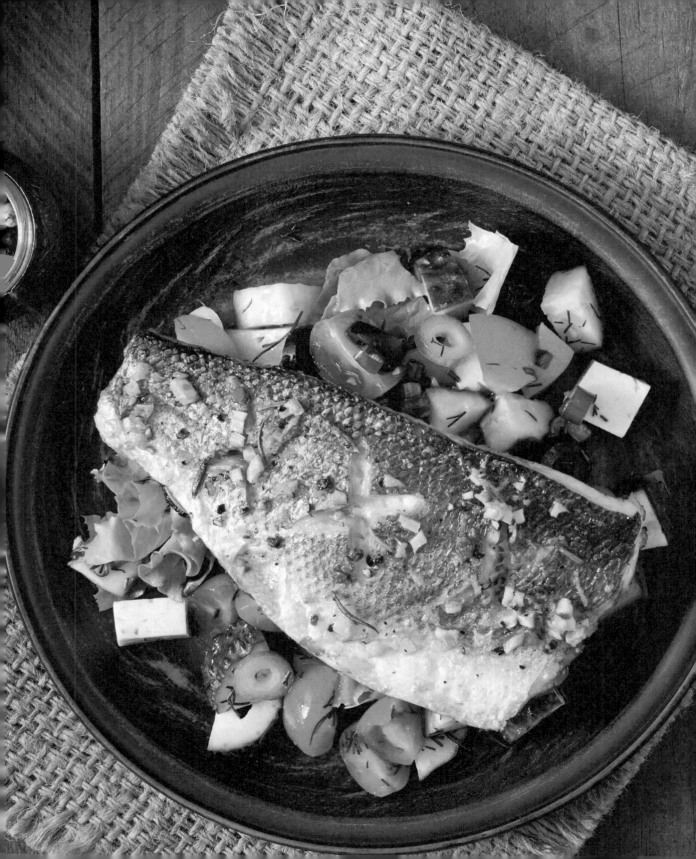

CHICKEN STIR-FRY WITH ASPARAGUS

 Cooking Difficulty: 3/10

 Cooking Time: 18 minutes

 Servings: 2

INGREDIENTS

- 2 chicken breasts
- 7 ounces asparagus
- 2 tablespoons soy sauce
- 1 tablespoon sesame oil
- 2 cloves garlic, minced
- 1 teaspoon fresh ginger, minced
- 1 teaspoon honey
- 2 tablespoons olive oil
- salt and pepper to taste
- sesame seeds for garnish (optional)

DESCRIPTION

STEP 1
Slice the chicken breasts into thin strips. Trim the ends of the asparagus and cut them into 2-inch pieces.

STEP 2
In a small bowl, mix together soy sauce, sesame oil, minced garlic, minced ginger, and honey.

STEP 3
On a preheated skillet, add olive oil. Then add the chicken and cook for 5 minutes. After that, add the asparagus and cook for another 3-4 minutes. Then add the sauce and cook until thickened. Garnish with sesame seeds.

NUTRITIONAL INFORMATION

Calories 364, Fat 12,3g, Carbs 16g, Protein 18g

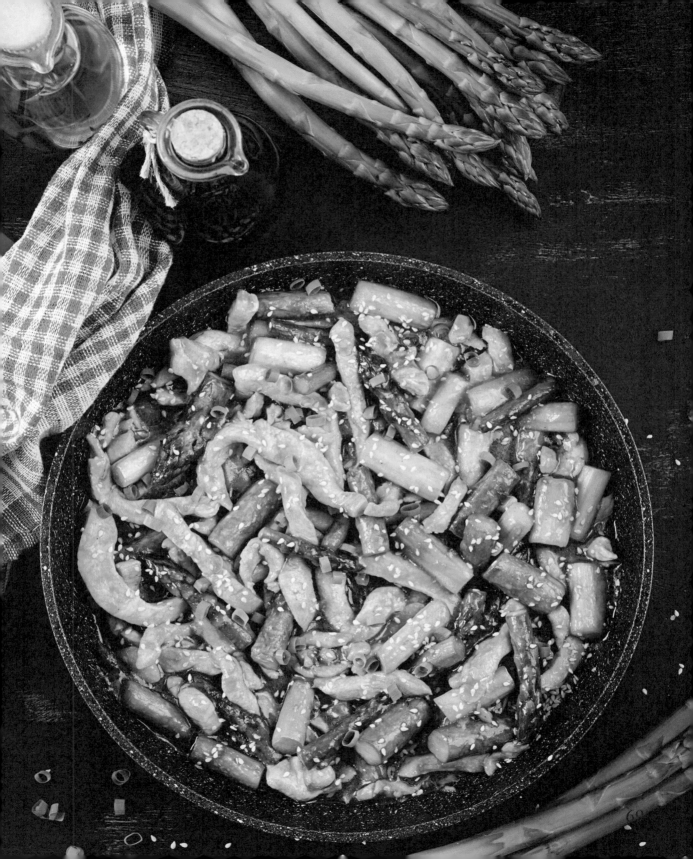

COCONUT CHICKPEA CURRY

 Cooking Difficulty: 4/10

 Cooking Time: 27 minutes

 Servings: 4

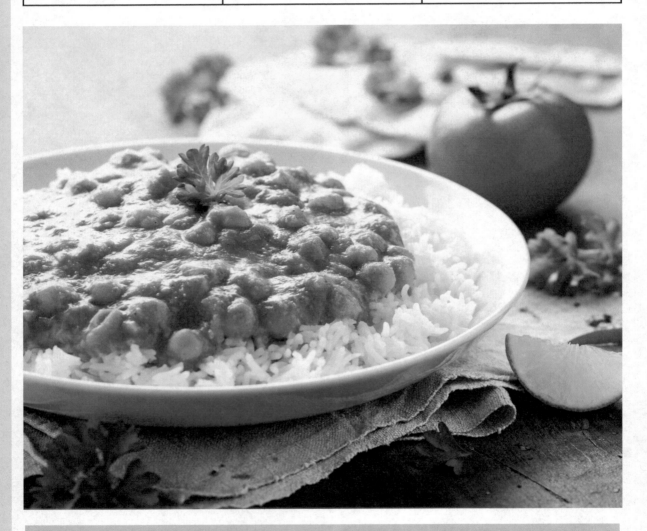

NUTRITIONAL INFORMATION

Calories: 225, Fat: 9.4 g, Carbs: 28.5 g, Protein: 7.3

INGREDIENTS

- 2 tsps. coconut flour
- 16 oz. cooked chickpeas
- 14 oz. tomatoes, diced
- 1 onion, sliced
- 1 ½ tsps. minced garlic
- ½ tsp. salt
- 1 tsp. curry powder
- 1/3 tsp. ground black pepper
- ¼ tsp. cumin
- 1 lemon, juiced
- 13.5 oz. coconut milk, unsweetened
- 2 tbsps. coconut oil

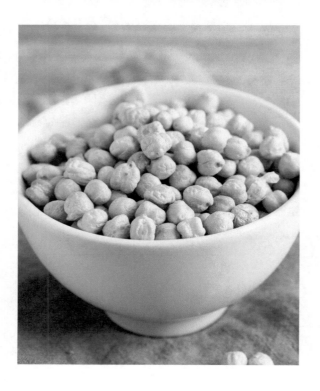

DESCRIPTION

STEP 1
Take a large pot, place it over medium-high heat, add oil and when it melts, add onions and tomatoes, season with salt and black pepper and cook for 5 minutes.

STEP 2
Switch heat to medium-low level, cook for 10 minutes until tomatoes have released their liquid, then add chickpeas and stir in garlic, curry powder, and cumin until combined.

STEP 3
Stir in milk and flour, bring the mixture to boil, then switch heat to medium heat and simmer the curry for 12 minutes until cooked.

STEP 4
Taste to adjust seasoning, drizzle with lemone juice, and serve. Place remaining portions in an airtight container and refrigerate for up to 2 days. Reheat before serving.

AVOCADO SALMON SALAD

 Cooking Difficulty: 1/10

 Cooking Time: 3 minutes

 Servings: 2

INGREDIENTS

- chopped lightly salted salmon
- 2 tbsp. avocado oil
- 2 sliced avocados
- 2 tbsp. lime juice
- 1 sliced cucumber
- black pepper
- favorite lettuce leaves if desired

DESCRIPTION

STEP 1

In a bowl, mix the avocado slices with the salmon and the rest of the ingredients, stir and serve for lunch.

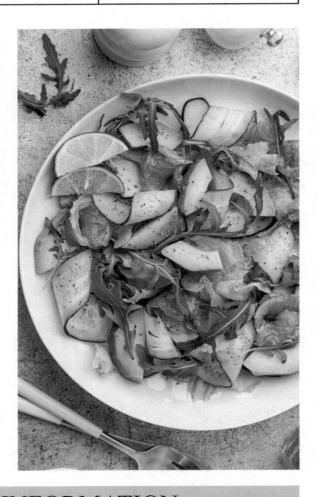

NUTRITIONAL INFORMATION

Calories 200, Fat 10g, Carbs 3g, Protein 7g

DELICIOUS SALMON

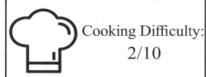 Cooking Difficulty: 2/10	Cooking Time: 16 minutes	Servings: 2

INGREDIENTS

- 2 salmon steak
- 1 tbsp. olive oil
- salt, pepper
- half a lemon
- salad leaves for serving

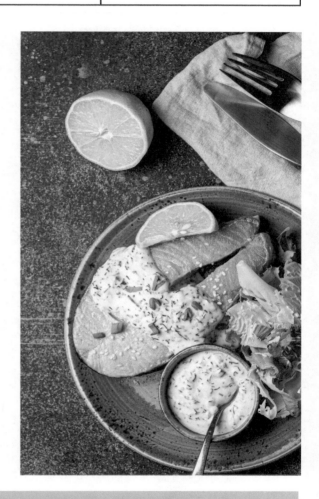

DESCRIPTION

STEP 1

Heat up a pan with the oil over medium-high heat. Add fish, salt, and pepper, cook for 4 minutes on each side, divide onto plates and serve with your favorite salad and lemon.

NUTRITIONAL INFORMATION

362 Calories, 7g Fats, 4.7g Carbs, 5.8 Protein

ZUCCHINI CAKES

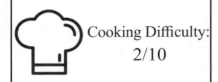 Cooking Difficulty: 2/10

 Cooking Time: 22 minutes

 Servings: 4

INGREDIENTS

- 2 tbsps. olive oil
- 2 tbsps. almond flour
- 1/3 c. carrot, shredded
- 1 tsp. lemon zest, grated
- 1 garlic clove, minced
- 1 egg, whisked
- 2 zucchinis, grated
- 1 yellow onion, chopped
- black pepper
- sea salt

DESCRIPTION

STEP 1

In a bowl, combine the zucchinis with the garlic, onion, and the other ingredients except for the oil, stir well and shape medium cakes out of this mix.

STEP 2

Heat up a pan with the oil over medium-high heat, add the zucchini cakes, cook for 5 minutes on each side, divide between plates and serve with a side salad.

NUTRITIONAL INFORMATION

Calories 271, Fat 8.7g, Carbs 14.3g, Protein 4.6g

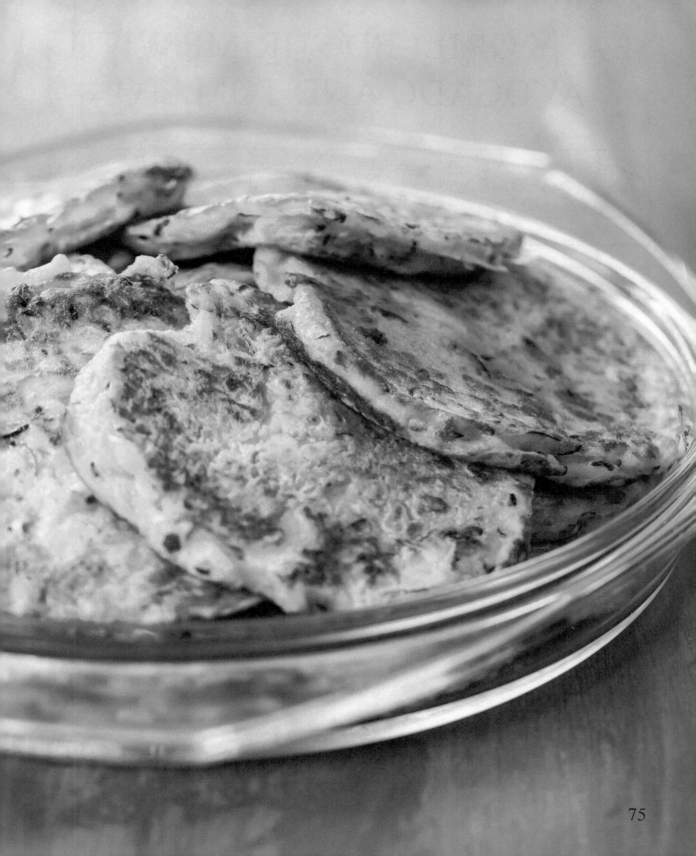

EASY GRILLED SHRIMP WITH AVOCADO AND TOMATO

 Cooking Difficulty: 3/10

 Cooking Time: 12 minutes

 Servings: 6

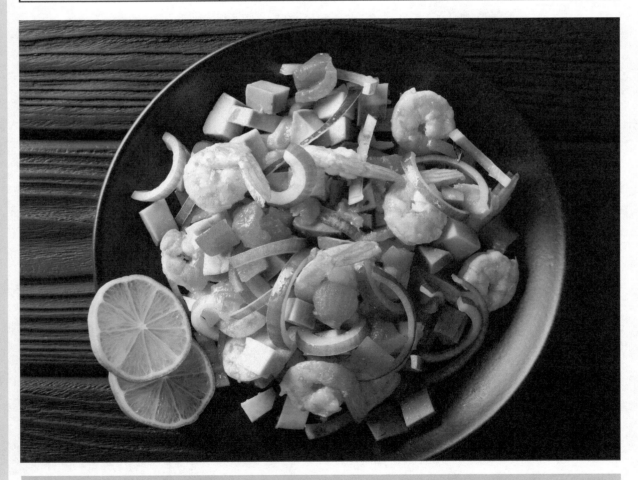

NUTRITIONAL INFORMATION

300 Calories, 11g Fats, 5g Carbs, 5g Protein

INGREDIENTS

- 2 cubed avocados
- 2 lb. deveined shrimp
- ½ c. chopped tomato
- ½ c. chopped bell pepper
- ½ c. chopped onion
- 4 tbsps. olive oil
- 2 tsps. squeezed lime juice
- 1 tsp. garlic powder
- 1 tsp. fine sea salt
- ¼ tsp. black pepper

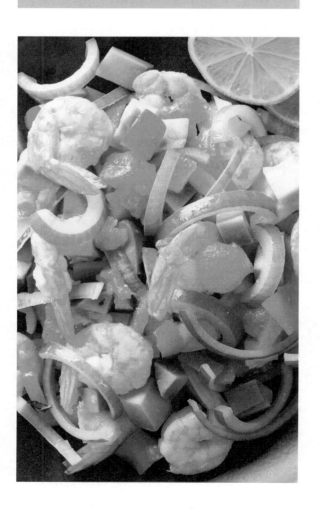

DESCRIPTION

STEP 1
Place a grill over medium-high flame and heat through.

STEP 2
Meanwhile, combine the garlic powder, half the salt and pepper, and olive oil in a large bowl. Add the shrimp and toss well to coat. Set aside.

STEP 3
In a salad bowl, combine the bell pepper, tomato, onion, avocado, and lime juice. Season with the remaining salt and toss gently to coat. Cover and refrigerate until ready to serve.

STEP 4
Cook the shrimp in the hot grill for 3 minutes per side, or until cooked through.

STEP 5
Divide the shrimp into individual servings, followed by the salad. Cover and refrigerate for up to 3 days. Reheat the shrimp before serving.

GINGER HALIBUT

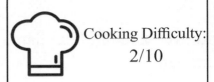 Cooking Difficulty: 2/10

 Cooking Time: 18 minutes

 Servings: 3

INGREDIENTS

- 24 oz. Alaskan halibut fillets
- 1½ tbsps. minced fresh ginger
- 1½ tsps. soy sauce
- 1½ tsps. olive oil
- ¾ tsp. rice wine vinegar

DESCRIPTION

STEP 1
Set the oven to 400 degrees F to preheat. Line a baking sheet with aluminum foil and set it aside.

STEP 2
Combine rice vinegar and olive oils in a bowl, then stir in the soy sauce, and ginger. Add the fish fillets and turn several times to coat.

STEP 3
Arrange the fish fillets on the prepared baking sheet—Bake for 17 minutes, or until done

NUTRITIONAL INFORMATION

380 Calories, 6g Fats, 3.4g Carbs, 7g Protein

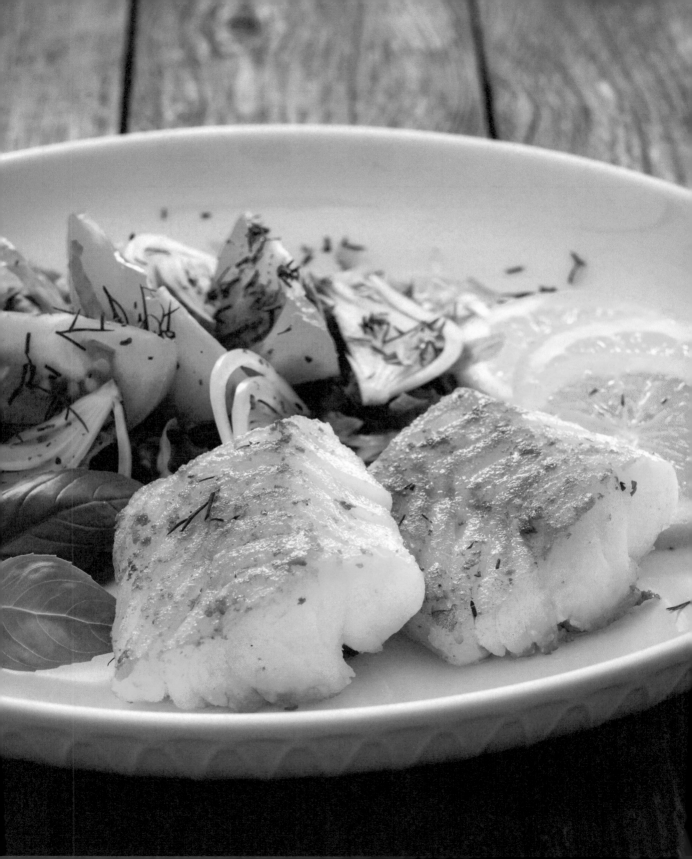

CHICKEN STEW

 Cooking Difficulty: 3/10

 Cooking Time: 23 minutes

 Servings: 4

INGREDIENTS

- 1 lb. cubed chicken breast, skinless and boneless
- 1 c. vegetable stock
- ½ c. tomato passata
- 1 chopped red onion
- 1 tbsp. olive oil
- 1 cubed red bell pepper
- 1 chopped shallot
- salt
- black pepper
- 3 minced garlic cloves
- 1 c. halved cherry tomatoes
- 1 tbsp. chopped cilantro

DESCRIPTION

STEP 1
Ensure that you heat the pan; add the shallot and the garlic and sauté for 2 minutes.

STEP 2
Add the meat and brown it for 3 minutes.

STEP 3
Add the stock and the other ingredients, bring to a simmer, then cook over medium heat for 15 minutes more, stirring from time to time.

STEP 4
Divide the stew into bowls and serve for dinner.

NUTRITIONAL INFORMATION

352 Calories, 17.2g Fats, 5.5g Carbs, 7.3g Protein

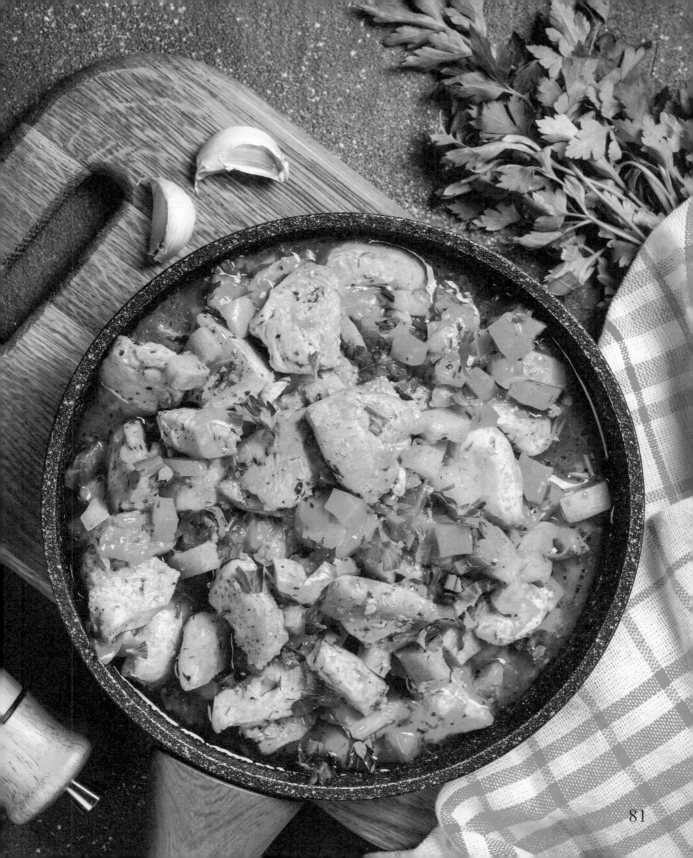

SPINACH WITH GARBANZO BEANS

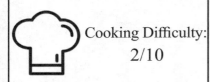 Cooking Difficulty:
2/10

 Cooking Time:
8 minutes

 Servings:
4

INGREDIENTS

- 1 tbsp. olive oil
- 4 minced garlic cloves
- ½ diced onion
- 10 oz. chopped spinach
- 12 oz. garbanzo beans
- ½ tsp. cumin
- ½ tsp. salt

DESCRIPTION

STEP 1
In a skillet, warm the olive oil over medium-low heat.

STEP 2
Then add the onions and garlic and cook until the onions are translucent. About 5 minutes.

STEP 3
Stir in spinach, cumin, salt, and garbanzo beans.

STEP 4
Allow cooking until thoroughly heated.

NUTRITIONAL INFORMATION

90 Calories, 4g Fat, 11g Carbs, 4g Protein

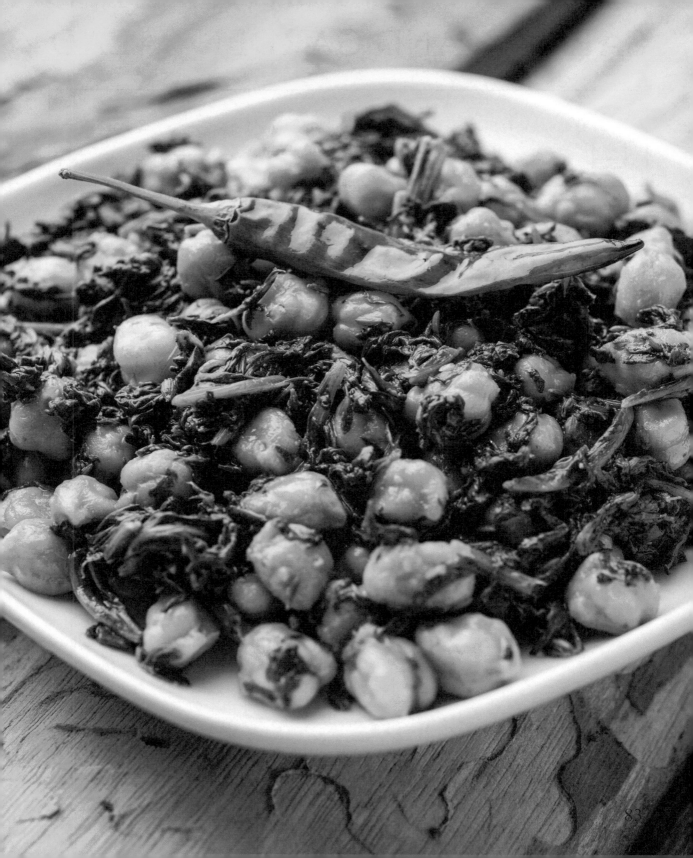

SARDINE AND GARDEN SALAD

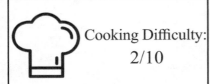 Cooking Difficulty: 2/10

 Cooking Time: 5 minutes

 Servings: 3

INGREDIENTS

- 1 diced cucumber
- 2 diced tomatoes
- 1 minced red onion
- 2 chopped sardine fillets
- 2 c. chopped arugula leaves
- ¼ c. chopped fresh flat-leaf parsley
  for the dressing:
- 2 tbsps. extra virgin olive oil
- ½ tbsp. squeezed lemon juice
- sea salt
- black pepper

DESCRIPTION

STEP 1
Combine the ingredients for the dressing in a bowl and set aside.

STEP 2
Toss together the chopped sardines, vegetables, and herbs in a bowl. Mix well, then divide into individual servings.

STEP 3
Divide the whole sardine fillets among the servings.

STEP 4
Drizzle the dressing over the salads, then cover and refrigerate for up to 3 days.

NUTRITIONAL INFORMATION

150 Calories, 19g Fats, 8g Carbs, and 6g Protein

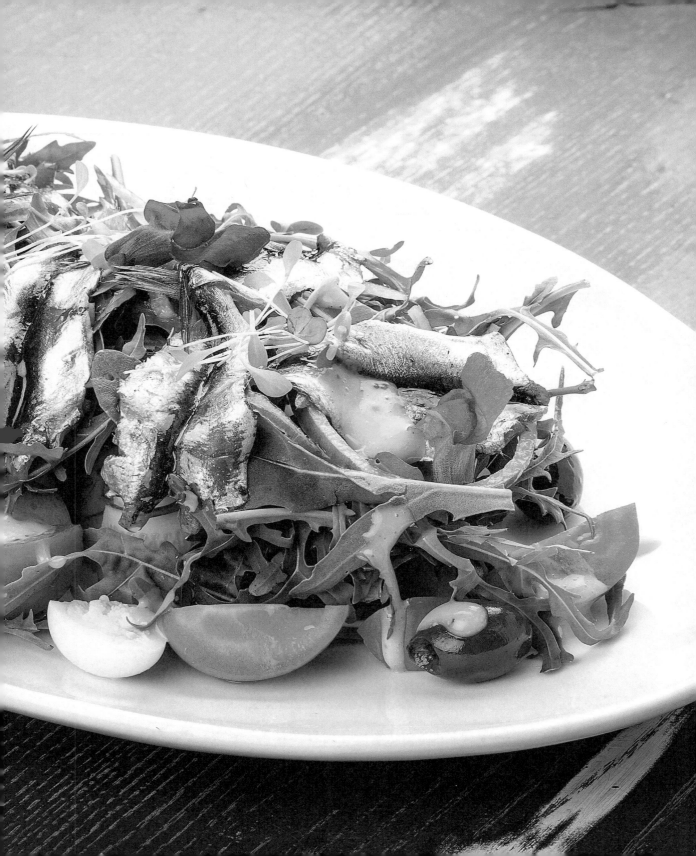

SEARED SALMON AND WHITE BEANS

 Cooking Difficulty: 3/10

 Cooking Time: 15 minutes

 Servings: 2

INGREDIENTS

- 8 oz. salmon fillet
- 1 medium tomato
- 1 the small bulb of fennel
- 15 oz. white beans
- 3 tsps. olive oil

- ¼ c. dry white wine
- 1½ tsps. dijon mustard
- 1 tsp. fennel seed
- ¼ tsp. pepper

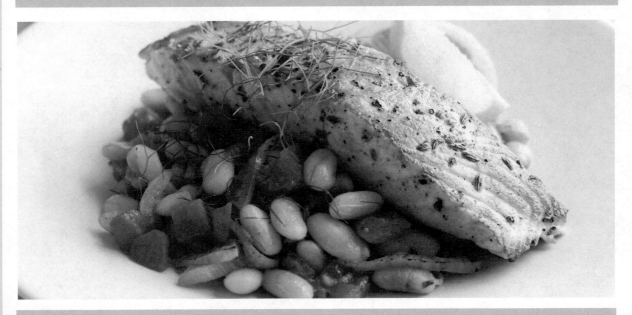

NUTRITIONAL INFORMATION

485 Calories, 23g Fat, 39g Carbs, 35g Protein

STEP 1

Begin by heating a tablespoon of olive oil in a large skillet over medium heat.

STEP 2

Add in the sliced fennel and cook for about 6 minutes or until lightly browned.

STEP 3

When this is done, stir in the white wine, tomato, and beans for about 3 minutes.

STEP 4

After the mixture is done cooking, transfer it into a bowl and stir in the chopped fennel, mustard, and a 1/8 teaspoon of pepper.

STEP 5

Before continuing, rinse and dry the pan you just used.

STEP 6

In a small bowl, combine the fennel seed and a 1/8 teaspoon of pepper, and then sprinkle the mixture on both sides of the salmon.

STEP 7

In the pan, heat up the remaining two teaspoons of olive oil over medium-high heat, and then add the salmon. Cook for 3-6 minutes or until golden brown. Be sure to cook both sides of the salmon.

STEP 8

Last, place the beans onto a plate and top with the salmon. Your meal is complete!

GRILLED CHICKEN BREAST

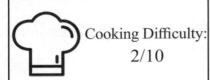 Cooking Difficulty: 2/10

 Cooking Time: 17 minutes

 Servings: 2

INGREDIENTS

- 2 chicken breasts
- 2 tablespoons olive oil
- 1 teaspoon salt
- 1/2 teaspoon black pepper
- 1/2 teaspoon turmeric
- 1/2 teaspoon cumin
- 1/2 teaspoon paprika
- 1/4 teaspoon garlic powder
- 1/4 teaspoon cayenne pepper (optional)

DESCRIPTION

STEP 1

In a bowl, mix together olive oil, salt, black pepper, turmeric, cumin, paprika, garlic powder, and cayenne pepper. Prepare the chicken breasts by trimming any excess fat and membranes. Rub the marinade onto each chicken breast, covering them evenly on both sides.

STEP 2

Preheat the grill to medium heat and brush it with oil to prevent sticking. Place the chicken breasts on the grill and cook for 6-7 minutes on each side, or until cooked through. Serve the grilled chicken breast with any fresh salad of your choice.

NUTRITIONAL INFORMATION

304 Calories, 9.9g Fat, 11.8g Carbs, 15.9g Protein

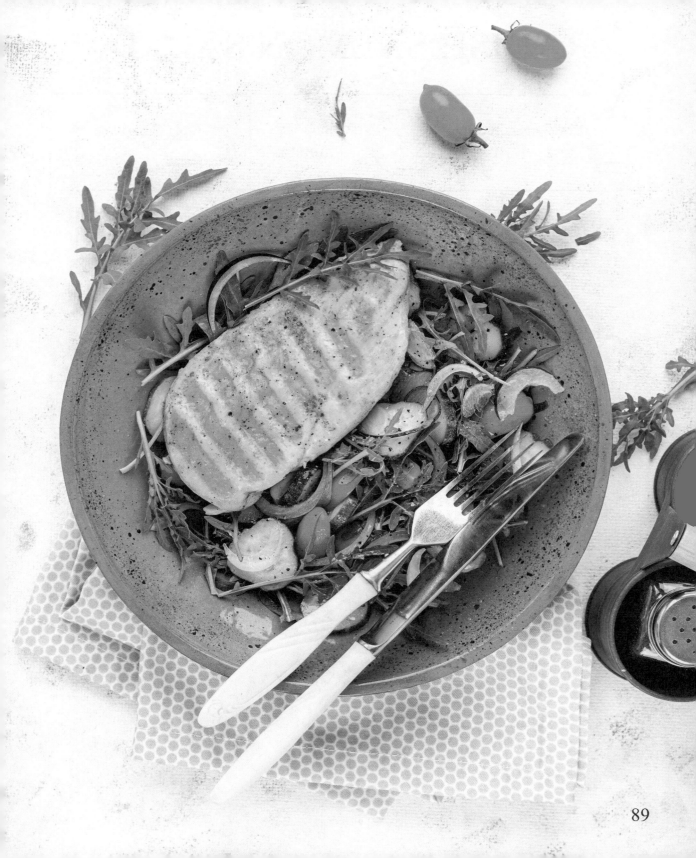

RADISH SALMON SALAD

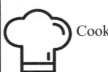 Cooking Difficulty: 1/10

 Cooking Time: 3 minutes

 Servings: 2

INGREDIENTS

- 1 grilled and sliced salmon steak
- 2 tablespoons olive oil
- 8 sliced radishes
- 2 tbsp. lemon juice
- black pepper, salt
- favorite lettuce leaves

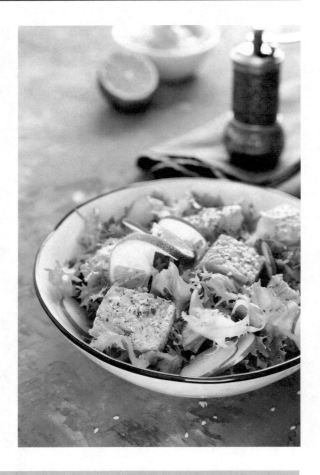

DESCRIPTION

STEP 1

In a bowl, mix the radishes slices with the salmon and the rest of the ingredients, stir and serve for lunch.

NUTRITIONAL INFORMATION

Calories 300, Fat 8g, Carbs 5g, Protein 6g

CUMIN SALMON

 Cooking Difficulty: 2/10

 Cooking Time: 7 minutes

 Servings: 4

INGREDIENTS

- 4 salmon fillets, boneless
- 1 tbsp. olive oil
- 1 sliced red onion
- salt
- black pepper
- 1 tsp. ground cumin

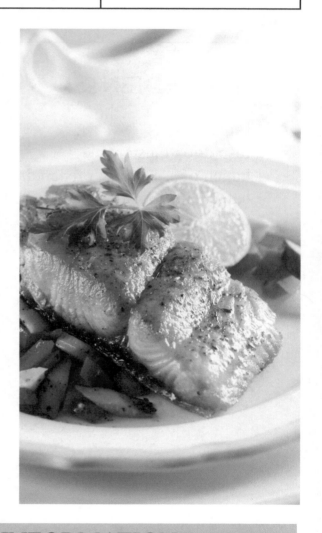

DESCRIPTION

STEP 1

Heat up a pan with the oil over medium-high heat, add the onion then cook for 2 minutes. Add the fish, salt, pepper, and the cumin, cook for 4 minutes on each side, divide between plates and serve.

NUTRITIONAL INFORMATION

Calories 300, Fat 14g, Carbs 5g, Protein 20g

DIJON MUSTARD GLAZED SALMON

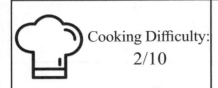 Cooking Difficulty: 2/10

 Cooking Time: 22 minutes

 Servings: 2

INGREDIENTS

- 2 salmon fillets
- 2 tbsp dijon mustard
- 1 bunch of asparagus, prepared
- 1 cup cherry tomatoes, halved
- 2 tbsp olive oil
- salt and black pepper to taste
- fresh lemon (optional)

DESCRIPTION

STEP 1
Preheat the oven to 400°F (200°C). Place the salmon fillets on a baking sheet lined with parchment paper. Brush each salmon fillet with Dijon mustard. Season with salt and black pepper to taste.

STEP 2
Bake the salmon in the preheated oven for 12-15 minutes or until done. In the last 5 minutes, add asparagus and tomatoes to the baking sheet, drizzle with olive oil.

STEP 3
Enjoy this light dish!

NUTRITIONAL INFORMATION
221 Calories, 11g Fat, 4g Carbs, 8g Protein

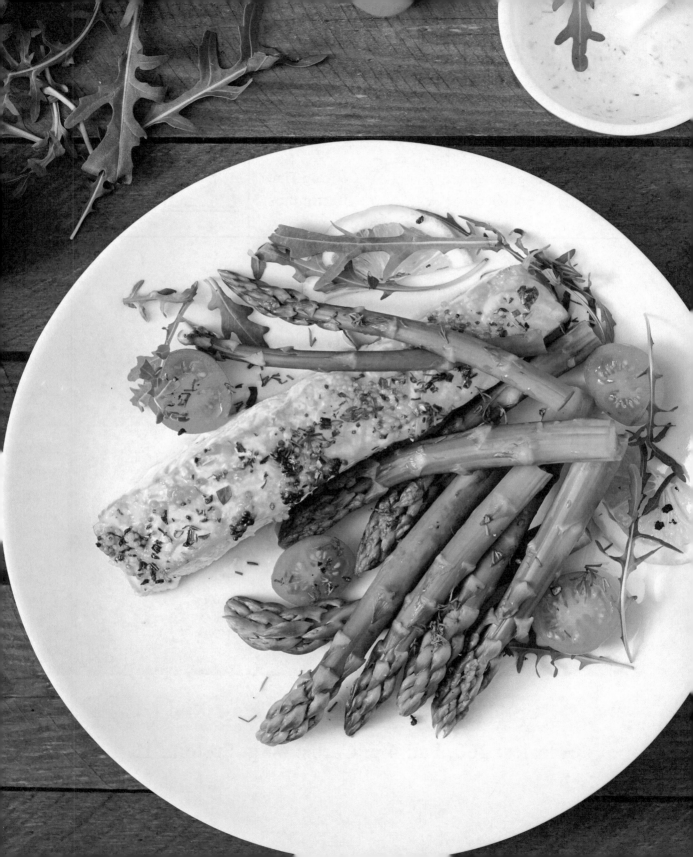

SWEET POTATO AND WHITE BEAN SKILLET

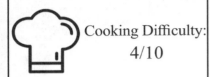 Cooking Difficulty: 4/10	Cooking Time: 30 minutes	Servings: 4

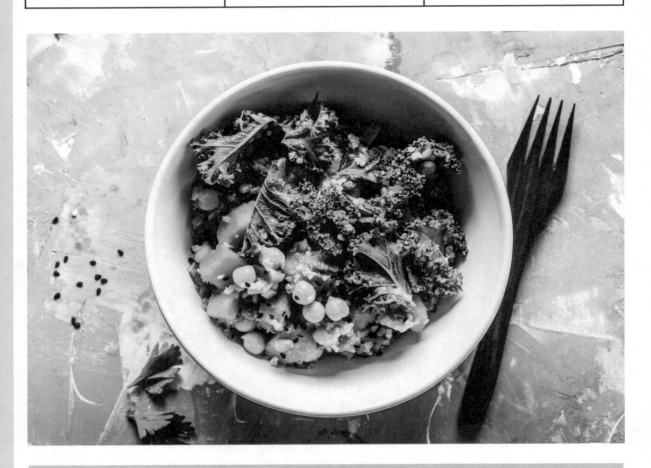

NUTRITIONAL INFORMATION

Calories: 260, Fat: 4 g, Carbs: 44 g, Protein: 13 g

INGREDIENTS

- 1 bunch kale, chopped
- 2 sweet potatoes, peeled, cubed
- 12 oz. cannellini beans
- 1 peeled onion, diced
- 1/8 tsp. red pepper flakes
- 1 tsp. salt
- ½ tsp. black pepper
- 1 tsp. curry powder
- 1 ½ tbsps. coconut oil
- 6 oz. coconut milk
- chickpeas (optional)

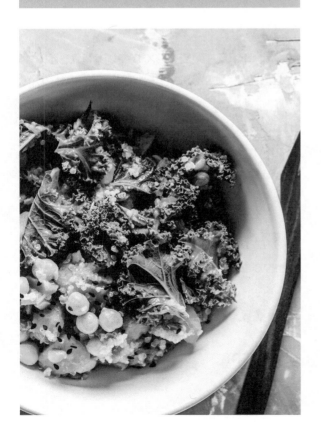

DESCRIPTION

STEP 1
Take a large skillet pan, place it over medium heat, add ½ tablespoon oil and when it melts, add onion and cook for 5 minutes.

STEP 2
Then stir in sweet potatoes, stir well, cook for 5 minutes, then season with all the spices, cook for 1 minute and remove the pan from heat.

STEP 3
Take another pan, add remaining oil in it, place it over medium heat and when oil melts, add kale, season with some salt and black pepper, stir well, pour in the milk and cook for 15 minutes until tender.

STEP 4
Then add beans, beans, and red pepper, stir until mixed and cook for 5 minutes until hot.

STEP 5
Serve straight away.

TUNA EGG SALAD

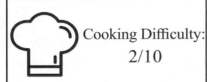 Cooking Difficulty: 2/10

 Cooking Time: 5 minutes

 Servings: 2

INGREDIENTS

- 1 can (about 150g) canned tuna, drained
- 2 tomatoes, diced
- salad leaves (of your choice), torn into pieces
- 1 cucumber, sliced
- 2 boiled eggs, sliced into wedges
- 1/2 red onion, thinly sliced
- 1 bunch of asparagus, trimmed and cooked
- 2 tablespoons olive oil
- salt and pepper to taste
- juice of half a lemon (optional)

DESCRIPTION

STEP 1
Drain the liquid from the canned tuna. Dice the tomatoes, slice the cucumber, boil and slice the eggs, and thinly slice the red onion.

STEP 2
In a large bowl, combine the tuna, tomatoes, salad leaves, cucumber, eggs, red onion, and cooked asparagus. Drizzle with olive oil. Season with salt and pepper to taste. Gently toss to ensure all ingredients are evenly distributed.

STEP 3
Serve and enjoy!

NUTRITIONAL INFORMATION

240 Calories, 23g Fat, 3g Carbs, 7g Protein

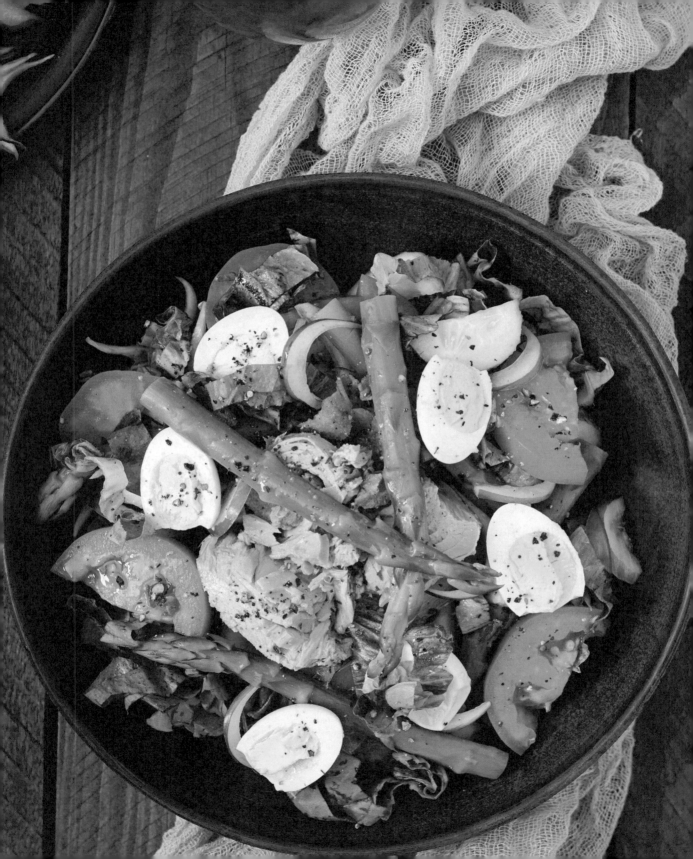

BAKED BROCCOLI

 Cooking Difficulty: 2/10

 Cooking Time: 20 minutes

 Servings: 4

INGREDIENTS

- 2 minced garlic cloves
- 2 tbsps. olive oil
- 1 lb. broccoli florets
- ½ tsp. ground nutmeg
- black pepper

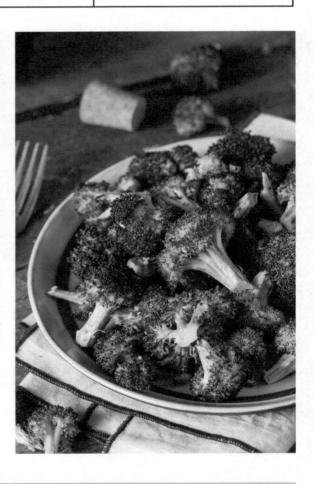

DESCRIPTION

STEP 1

In a roasting pan, combine the broccoli with the garlic and the other ingredients, toss and bake at 400 degrees F for 20 minutes. Divide the mix between plates and serve.

NUTRITIONAL INFORMATION

165 Calories, 8g Fats, 7g Carbs, 7g Protein

VEGETABLE WRAPS

 Cooking Difficulty: 2/10

 Cooking Time: 9 minutes

 Servings: 4

INGREDIENTS

- 1 head of romaine lettuce
- 2 carrots
- 1 cucumber
- 1 red onion
- 1 celery stalk
- dressing of choice

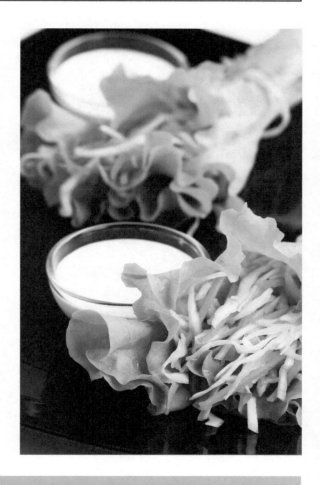

DESCRIPTION

STEP 1

Finely slice the carrots, cucumber, red onion, and celery into sticks of vegetable. Divide between 12 lettuce leaves. Roll up lettuce leaves and serve.

NUTRITIONAL INFORMATION

20 Calories, 6g Fats, 1g Carbs, and 0g Protein

ITALIAN TOMATO SOUP

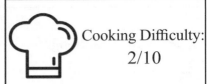 Cooking Difficulty: 2/10

 Cooking Time: 25 minutes

 Servings: 3

INGREDIENTS

- 1 pound tomatoes
- 3 cloves of garlic
- 3 cups vegetable broth
- 2 tbsp. olive oil
- 1 green basil, bundle
- dry bread (optional)
- sea salt
- black pepper

DESCRIPTION

STEP 1
Heat olive oil in a large saucepan over medium heat. Add the garlic and fry for 1 minute.

STEP 2
In a separate bowl, chop the tomatoes. Place them in the pan. Season with salt and pepper. Partially cover and stew over medium heat for about ten minutes. Add the broth and basil, return to the stove and simmer for another ten minutes. Add the bread cubes and stew for another ten minutes until the bread is soft.

STEP 3
Serve with extra olive oil and put in more fresh basil!

NUTRITIONAL INFORMATION

110 Calories, 2g Fats, 3g Carbs, and 3g Protein

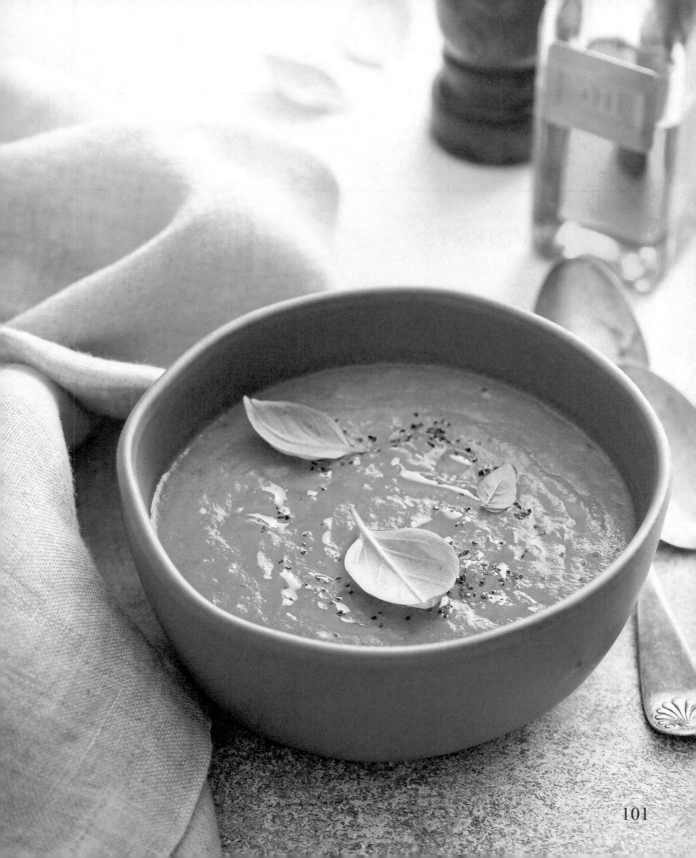

TERIYAKI CHICKEN

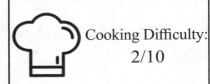 Cooking Difficulty: 2/10

 Cooking Time: 20 minutes

 Servings: 2

INGREDIENTS

- 1 chicken filet
- 2 spoons of teriyaki sauce
- 1 spoonful of soy sauce
- green onions for decoration

DESCRIPTION

STEP 1
Cut the chicken fillet into small slices.

STEP 2
Heat a frying pan. Add the chicken to the pan and stir-fry. When the chicken is almost done, add the two sauces. Sauté the chicken so all the moisture is gone and the glaze comes out.

STEP 3
Serve with green onions and rice.

NUTRITIONAL INFORMATION

411 Calories, 11g Fats, 6g Carbs, 4.8 Protein

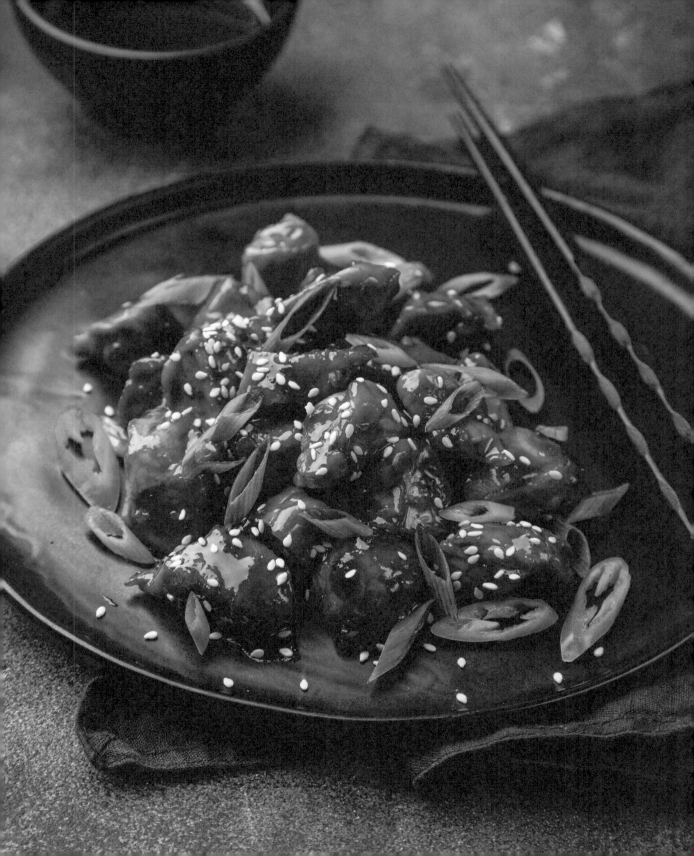

CHIPOTLE CHICKEN IN LETTUCE WRAPS

Cooking Difficulty: 3/10	Cooking Time: 30 minutes	Servings: 2

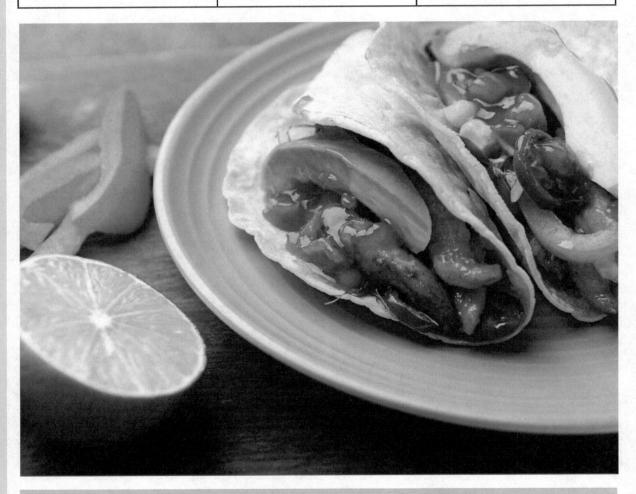

NUTRITIONAL INFORMATION

498 Calories, 27g Fats, 7g Carbs, 8 Protein

INGREDIENTS

- 2 tbsps. olive oil
- 400g tomatoes
- 400g skinless chicken breast
- 1 sliced red onion
- 1 tbsp. chopped chipotle in adobo sauce
- salt
- pepper
- ½ tsp. cumin
- lettuce leaves
- coriander leaves
- avocado slices
- lime wedges
- lime juice
  rustic salsa:
- cherry tomatoes
- sliced red onions
- scallions
- salt

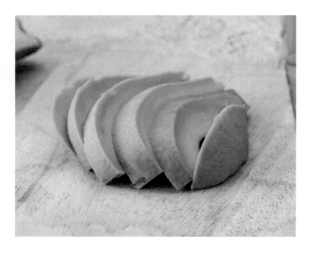

DESCRIPTION

STEP 1
Set oven to medium-high. Heat a nonstick frying pan and add the olive oil. Fry chicken pieces until golden brown. Put aside.

STEP 2
Add more olive oil to the same pan and fry the onion until it softens.

STEP 3
Add cumin, chipotle, tomatoes, and cumin and simmer for around 15 to 25 mins until the tomato sauce thickens on the pan edges.

STEP 4
Add the chicken back in the sauce and cook for 5 mins.

STEP 5
Arrange the ingredients to make your tacos in another bowl and serve. You can sprinkle lime juice to improve the flavor.

105

MUSHROOM SOUP

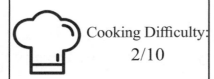 Cooking Difficulty: 2/10

 Cooking Time: 20 minutes

 Servings: 2

INGREDIENTS

- 1 pound champignons
- 3 shallots
- 2 cloves of garlic
- 2 cups chicken broth
- 7 tbsp. natural yogurt
- 2 tbsp. olive oil

DESCRIPTION

STEP 1
Sauté the finely chopped onion in a saucepan in olive oil until tender.

STEP 2
Add mushrooms and garlic. Then pour chicken broth into a saucepan, bring to a boil and cook for another 10 minutes, until mushrooms are tender.

STEP 3
Whisk the soup with a blender and season with natural yogurt before serving.

NUTRITIONAL INFORMATION

201 Calories, 8.1g Fats, 3g Carbs, 3 Protein

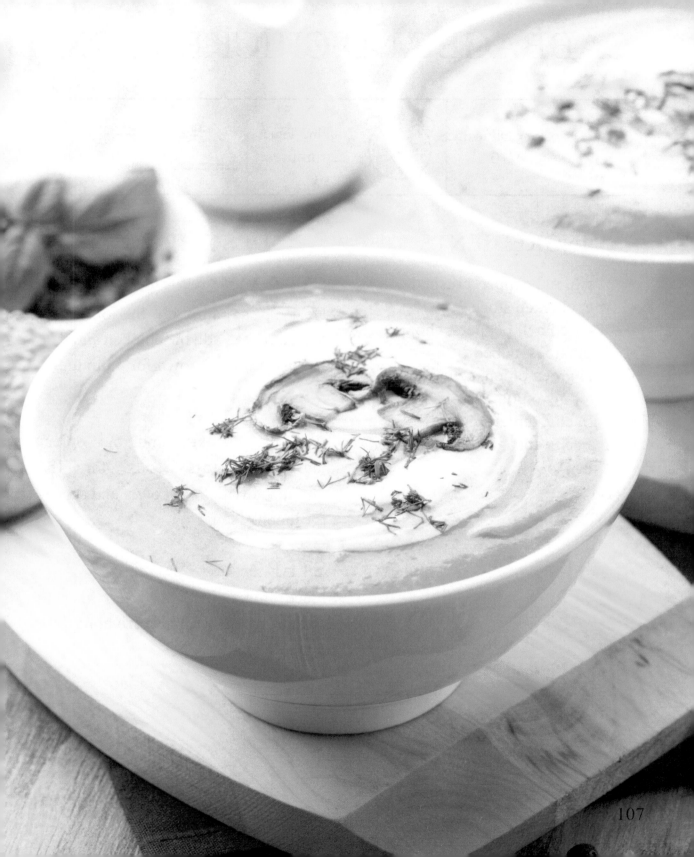

CABBAGE AND CHICKEN MIX

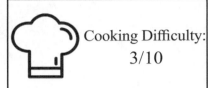 Cooking Difficulty: 3/10

 Cooking Time: 22 minutes

 Servings: 4

INGREDIENTS

- ¼ tsp. red pepper, crushed
- ¼ c. chicken stock
- ¾ c. red bell peppers, chopped
- 3 tomatoes, cubed
- ¼ c. green onions, chopped
- 1 yellow onion, chopped
- 1 lb. chicken ground
- 1 green cabbage head, shredded
- 1 tbsp. olive oil
- salt
- pepper

DESCRIPTION

STEP 1
Heat up a pan with the oil over medium heat, add the chicken and the onions, stir and brown for 5 minutes.

STEP 2
Add the cabbage and the other ingredients, toss, cook for 15 minutes, divide into bowls and serve for lunch.

STEP 2
Place remaining portions in an airtight container and refrigerate for up to 3 days.

NUTRITIONAL INFORMATION

340 Calories, 10g Fats, 4g Carbs, 4.9 Protein

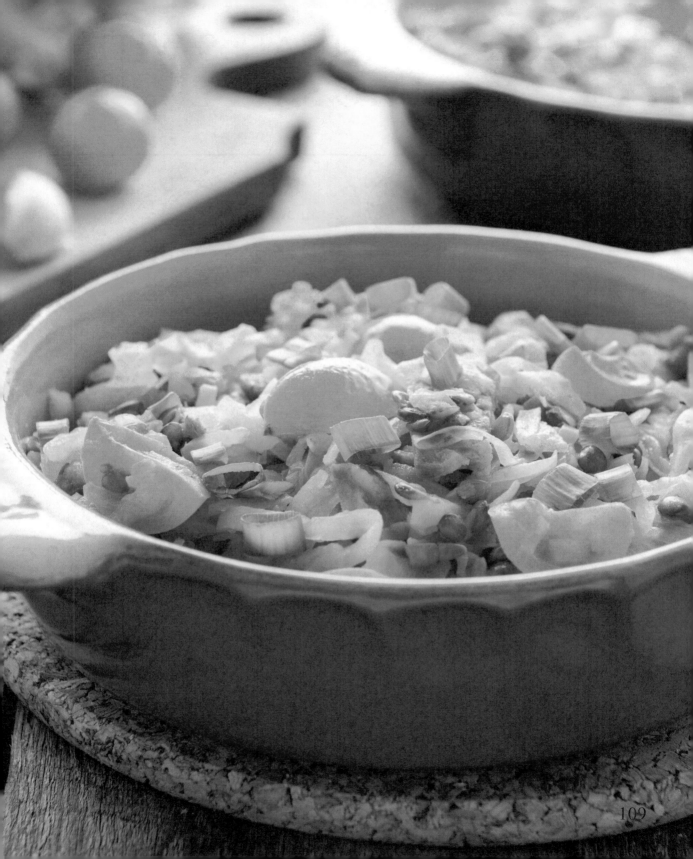

TURKEY MEATBALLS WITH TOMATO SAUCE

 Cooking Difficulty: 3/10

 Cooking Time: 25 minutes

 Servings: 4

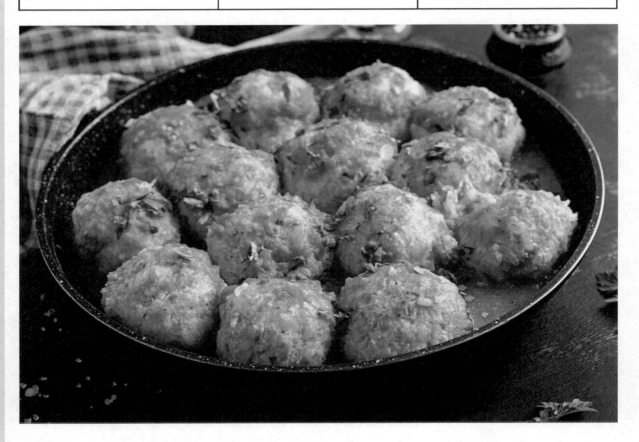

NUTRITIONAL INFORMATION

380 Calories, 26g Fats, 5g Carbs, 8g Protein

INGREDIENTS

- 7 oz. chopped fresh mushrooms
- 1 chopped onion
- 1 lightly beaten egg
- 1 tbsp. italian seasoning
- 14.5 oz. diced tomatoes
- 2 lb. lean ground turkey
- 2 tbsps. olive oil

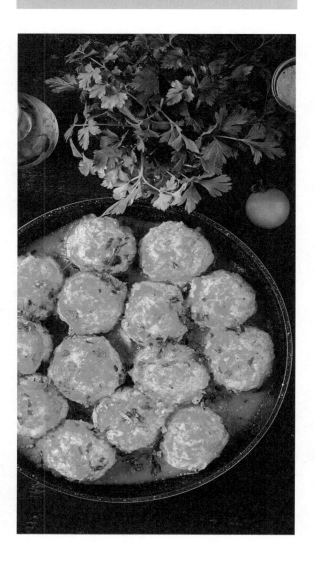

DESCRIPTION

STEP 1
In a medium-size bowl, combine mushrooms, egg, ground turkey, onion and Italian seasoning. Shape the mixture into meatballs.

STEP 2
Heat a nonstick skillet over medium heat. Add oil. Cook meatballs until brown, and there is no pink in the center or for four minutes with frequent stirring.

STEP 3
Remove from the pan and keep warm. Add tomatoes into the pan, let it boil, and simmer for 15 mins. or until thickens.

STEP 4
Add the cooked meatballs into the pan with tomatoes and simmer for around 5 minutes or until heated through.

BAKED VEGETABLES

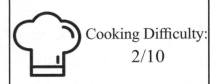 Cooking Difficulty: 2/10

 Cooking Time: 35 minutes

 Servings: 2

INGREDIENTS

- 2 minced garlic cloves
- 2 tablespoons olive oil
- 1/2 pound broccoli florets
- 2 carrots
- green beans (optional)
- black pepper
- salt
- 2 eggs

DESCRIPTION

STEP 1
Slice the carrots into slices. In a roasting pan, combine the vegetables together with the oil, garlic and spices, toss and bake at 400 degrees F for 15 minutes.

STEP 2
When the time is up, take out the mold and pour the two eggs into it. Return to the oven and bake until the eggs are cooked.

STEP 3
Divide the mix between plates and serve.

NUTRITIONAL INFORMATION

260 Calories, 4.9g Protein, 7g Fat, 4,4g Carbs

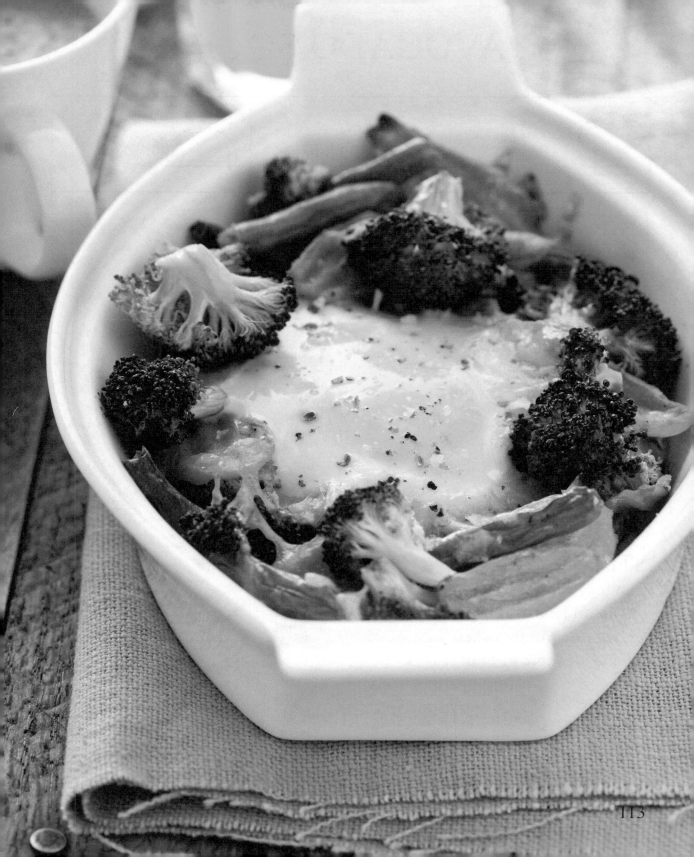

AVOCADO SOUP

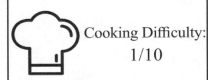 Cooking Difficulty: 1/10

 Cooking Time: 5 minutes

 Servings: 4

INGREDIENTS

- 2 pcs. avocado
- ½ pack of arugula
- mint handful
- ⅓ glasses of coconut cream
- 3.5 cups water
- 1 pc. lemon juice
- 1 tbsp. olive oil
- salt pepper

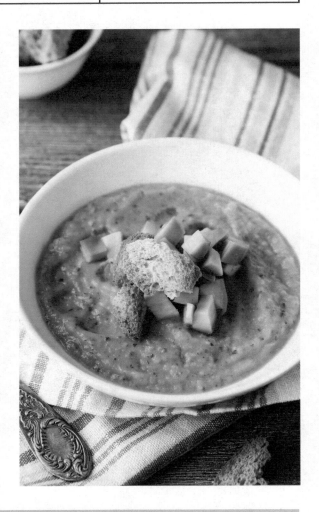

DESCRIPTION

STEP 1

Combine all ingredients (except oil) in a blender at high speed until smooth. Serve garnished with olive oil and a couple of mint leaves.

NUTRITIONAL INFORMATION

365 Calories, 22g Fats, 7g Carbs, 7g Protein

BEAN AND QUINOA SALAD

 Cooking Difficulty: 2/10

 Cooking Time: 5 minutes

 Servings: 10

INGREDIENTS

- 15 ounces boiled black beans
- 1 chopped red bell pepper without core
- 1 in. quinoa, cooked
- 1 green bell pepper, cored, chopped
- 5 ounces of canned corn
- parsley

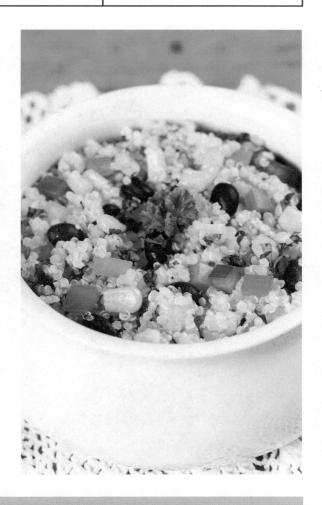

DESCRIPTION

STEP 1

In a bowl, set in all ingredients, and stir until incorporated. Top the salad with parsley and serve straight away.

NUTRITIONAL INFORMATION

Calories: 64, Fat: 1 g, Carbs: 8 g, Protein: 3 g

CHICKEN PIECES

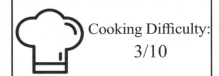 Cooking Difficulty: 3/10

 Cooking Time: 15 minutes

 Servings: 6

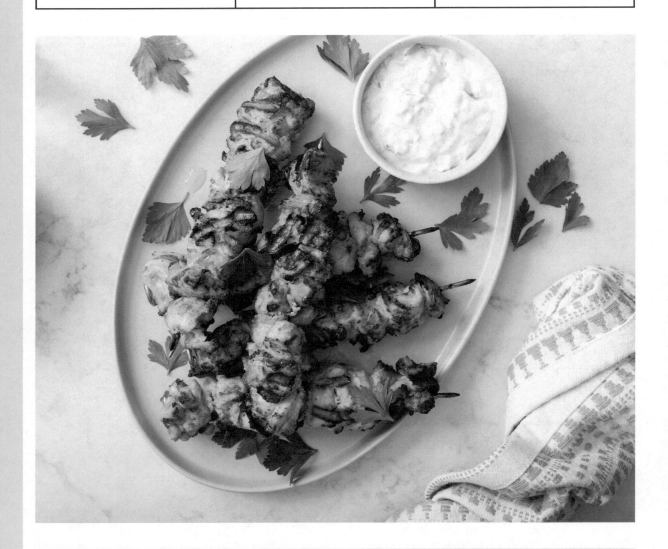

NUTRITIONAL INFORMATION

294 Calories, 5.2g Fat, 42.1g Carbs, 22.2g Protein

INGREDIENTS

- 2 tbsps. lemon juice
- 14 oz. greek yogurt
- 2 tsps. chopped oregano leaves
- ¼ c. white dry wine
- ¼ c. olive oil
- ½ tsp. pepper - divided
- 1 tsp. salt
- 2 lb. skinned breasts
- 4 minced garlic cloves
- 2 tsps. distilled white vinegar
- ½ c. cucumber

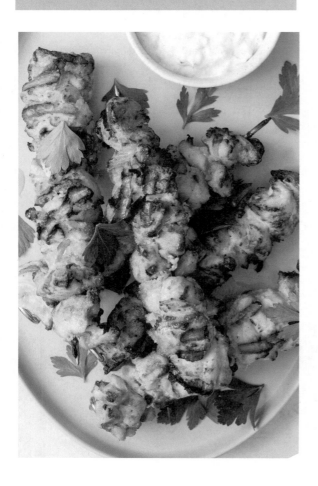

DESCRIPTION

STEP 1
Cut the chicken into ½-inch cubes, and coarsely shred the cucumber.

STEP 2
Set the grill between 450°F and 550°F.

STEP 3
Blend the wine, oil, chicken, oregano, lime juice, ¼ teaspoon of pepper, and salt in a mixing bowl.

STEP 4
Use eight metal skewers to prepare the chicken for cooking. Grill for approximately 10-12 minutes.

STEP 5
Remove any excess moisture from the cucumbers with paper towels, and put them into a medium dish. Mix in the yogurt, garlic, vinegar, and pepper with the cucumbers.

STEP 6
Serve with warm pita bread and chicken. Place remaining portions in an airtight container and refrigerate for up to 3 days.

BAKED CHICKEN WITH SWEET PAPRIKA

 Cooking Difficulty: 2/10

 Cooking Time: 35 minutes

 Servings: 4

INGREDIENTS

- 4 chicken fillets
- 2 tbsp. sweet paprika
- 3 tbsp. olive oil
- 3 tbsp. dried garlic
- salt
- black pepper

DESCRIPTION

STEP 1
Preheat oven to 380 F.

STEP 2
Rub the chicken fillet with spices and olive oil and let sit for 5 minutes.

STEP 3
Place the chicken in the oven and bake for 30 minutes.

STEP 4
Serve with salad or chopped vegetables.

NUTRITIONAL INFORMATION

Calories 298, Fat 9,3g, Carbs 6g, Protein 11g

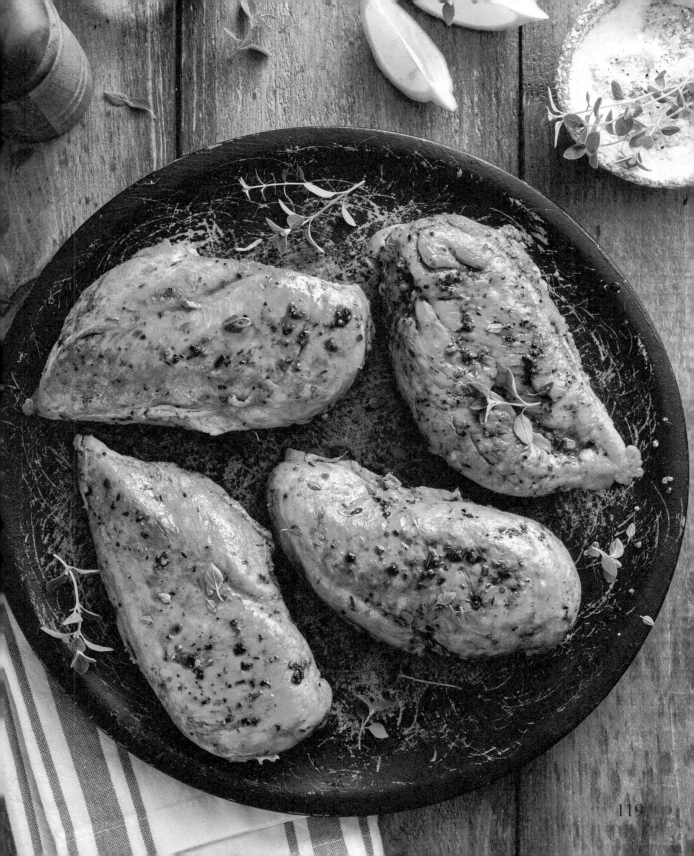

CHICKPEA AND SPINACH CUTLETS

Cooking Difficulty: 3/10	Cooking Time: 40 minutes	Servings: 12

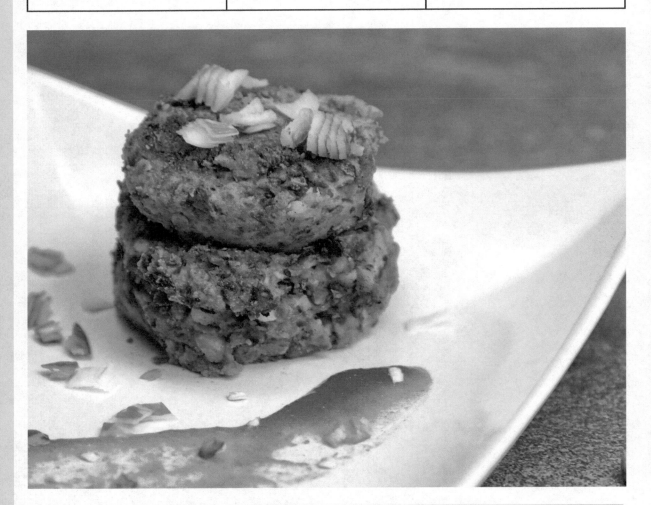

NUTRITIONAL INFORMATION

170 Calories, 5g Fat, 1.7g Carbs, 4g Protein

INGREDIENTS

- 1 red bell pepper
- 19 oz. chickpeas, rinsed & drained
- 1 c. ground almonds
- 2 tsps. dijon mustard
- 1 tsp. oregano
- 1 c. spinach, fresh
- 1½ c. rolled oats
- 1 clove garlic, pressed
- ½ lemon, juiced

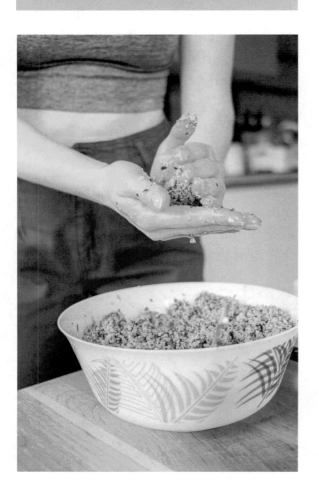

DESCRIPTION

STEP 1
Get out a baking sheet. Line it with parchment paper.

STEP 2
Cut your red pepper in half and then take the seeds out. Place it on your baking sheet, and roast it in the oven while you prepare your other ingredients.

STEP 3
Process your chickpeas, almonds, and mustard together in a food processor.

STEP 4
Add in your lemon juice, oregano, sage, garlic, and spinach, processing again. Make sure it's combined, but don't puree it.

STEP 5
Once your red bell pepper is softened, which should roughly take ten minutes, add this to the processor as well. Add in your oats, mixing well.

STEP 6
Form twelve patties, cooking in the oven for a half hour. They should be browned.

SAUTÉED GREEN BEANS WITH MACADAMIA NUTS

 Cooking Difficulty: 2/10

 Cooking Time: 15 minutes

 Servings: 2

INGREDIENTS

- 7 ounces (about 200g) green beans, trimmed and cut into bite-sized pieces
- 1/4 cup macadamia nuts, roughly chopped
- 1 tablespoon olive oil
- salt and pepper to taste
- optional: fresh lemon wedges and chopped parsley for garnish

DESCRIPTION

STEP 1
Heat olive oil in a skillet over medium heat. Add the green beans to the skillet and sauté, stirring occasionally, for about 5-7 minutes or until the beans are tender and lightly browned.

STEP 2
Next, add the chopped macadamia nuts to the skillet and sauté for an additional 2-3 minutes until they are fragrant and lightly toasted.

STEP 3
Season the sautéed green beans and macadamia nuts with salt and pepper to taste.

NUTRITIONAL INFORMATION

210 Calories, 4.9g Protein, 9g Fat, 8,4g Carbs

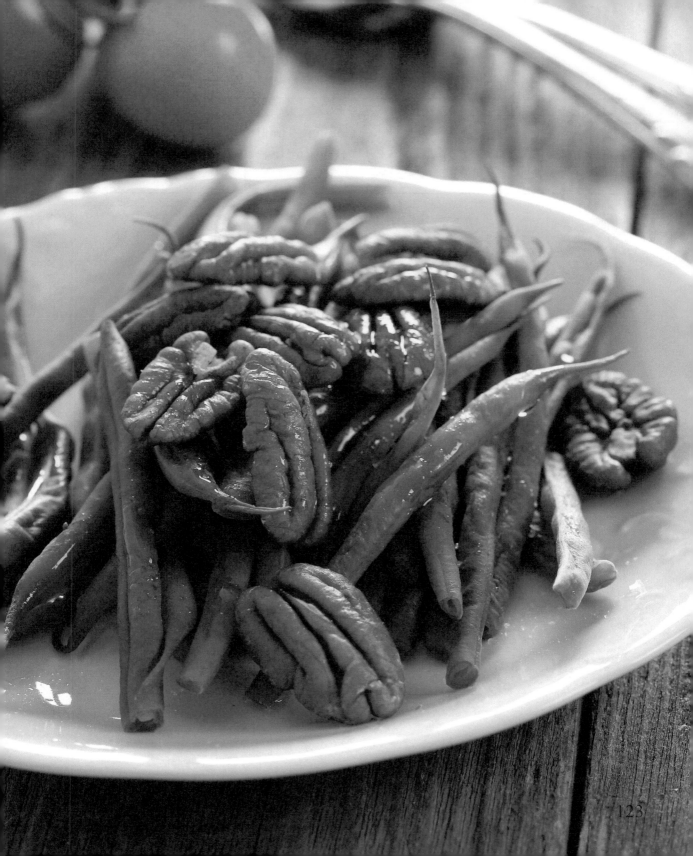

FISH TACOS

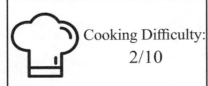 Cooking Difficulty:
2/10

 Cooking Time:
10 minutes

 Servings:
2

INGREDIENTS

- 1 tbsp. tomato puree
- 1 tbsp. salsa
- 1 tbsp. light mayonnaise
- 2 cod fillets, de-boned, skinless, and cubed
- 1 tbsp. coconut oil
- 1 tbsp. cilantro, chopped
- 4 taco shells, whole wheat
- 1 red onion, chopped

DESCRIPTION

STEP 1
Heat up a pan with the oil over medium heat, add the onion, stir and cook for 2 minutes.

STEP 2
Add the fish and tomato puree, toss gently, and cook for 5 minutes more.

STEP 3
Spoon this into the taco shells, also divide the mayo, salsa, and serve for lunch.

NUTRITIONAL INFORMATION

Calories 466, Fat 14.5g, Carbs 56.6g, Protein 32.9g

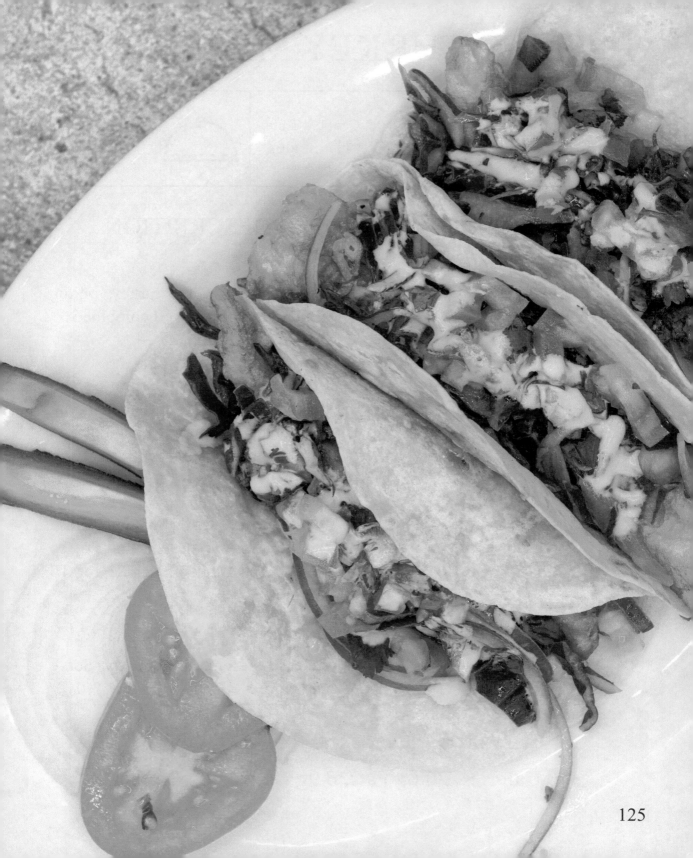

TOMATO TURKEY MEATBALLS

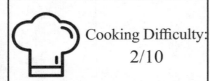 Cooking Difficulty: 2/10

 Cooking Time: 11 minutes

 Servings: 4

INGREDIENTS

- ground turkey, 1 lb.
- diced onion, ¼
- almond flour, 1/3 c.
- garlic powder, ½ tsp.
- chicken stock, ¼ c.
- diced tomatoes, 28 oz.
- olive oil, 1 tbsp.
- basil, ½ tsp.
- pepper, ¼ tsp.

DESCRIPTION

STEP 1
In a bowl, mix the turkey, onion, almond flour until well combined.

STEP 2
Shape the mixture into small meatballs. Place the remaining ingredients in your Instant Pot and stir to combine.

STEP 3
Place the meatballs inside. Close the lid and set the Instant Pot to MANUAL. Cook on HIGH for 10 minutes.

STEP 4
Release the pressure quickly. Serve and enjoy!

NUTRITIONAL INFORMATION

350 Calories, 20.6g Fats, 6.9g Carbs, 38g Protein

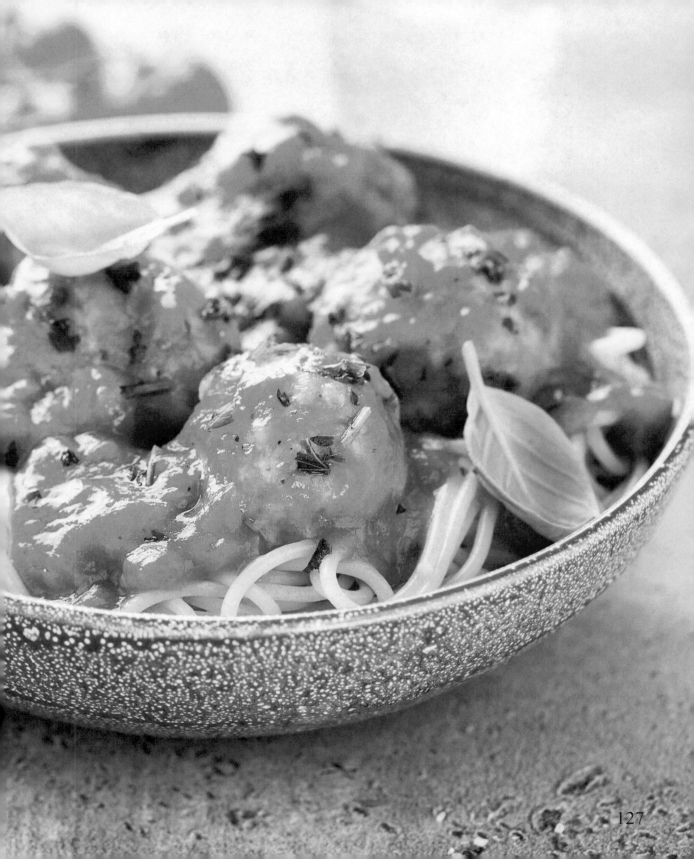

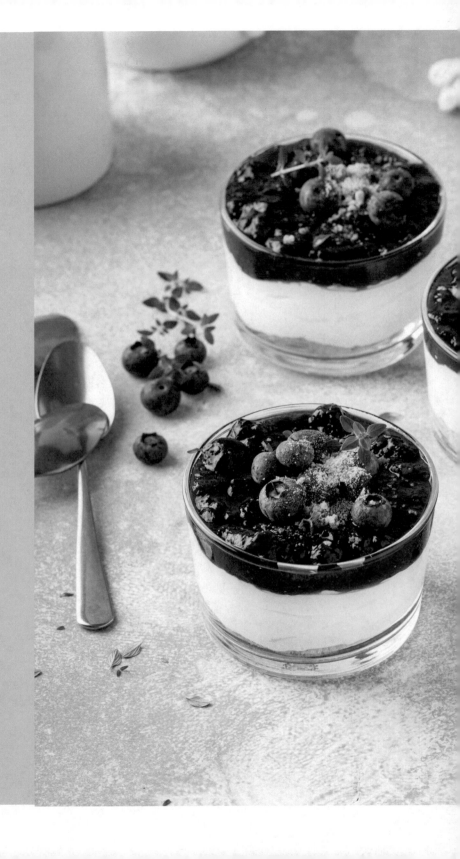

SNACKS & DESSERTS

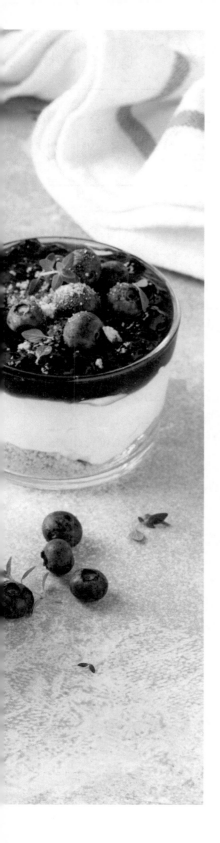

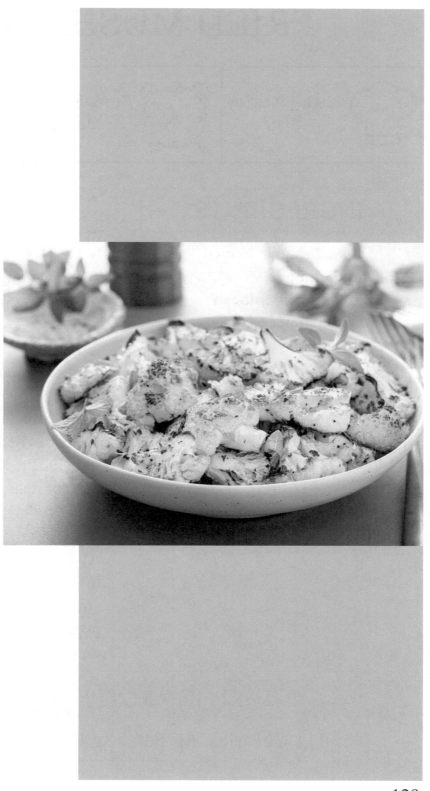

FRIED MUSHROOMS

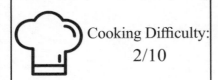 Cooking Difficulty: 2/10

 Cooking Time: 23 minutes

 Servings: 3

INGREDIENTS

- 1 lb mushrooms, halved
- 1 large onion
- 2 cloves garlic minced
- salt and pepper to taste
- 2 tablespoons of olive oil
- 1 tablespoon Worcestershire Sauce (optional)
- parsley
- italian herbs (optional)

DESCRIPTION

STEP 1
Heat a frying pan and add olive oil to it. Pour in the Worcestershire sauce.

STEP 2
Add the mushrooms and cook until golden brown, about 5 minutes. Add the onions and cook until the edges are browned and the onions are translucent. Stir in the mushrooms as they roast.

STEP 3
At the last minute, reduce the heat to low and add the crushed garlic, stirring continuously. Salt and pepper to taste. Garnish with parsley and serve.

NUTRITIONAL INFORMATION

111 Calories, 6g Fats, 3g Carbs, 6.8 Protein

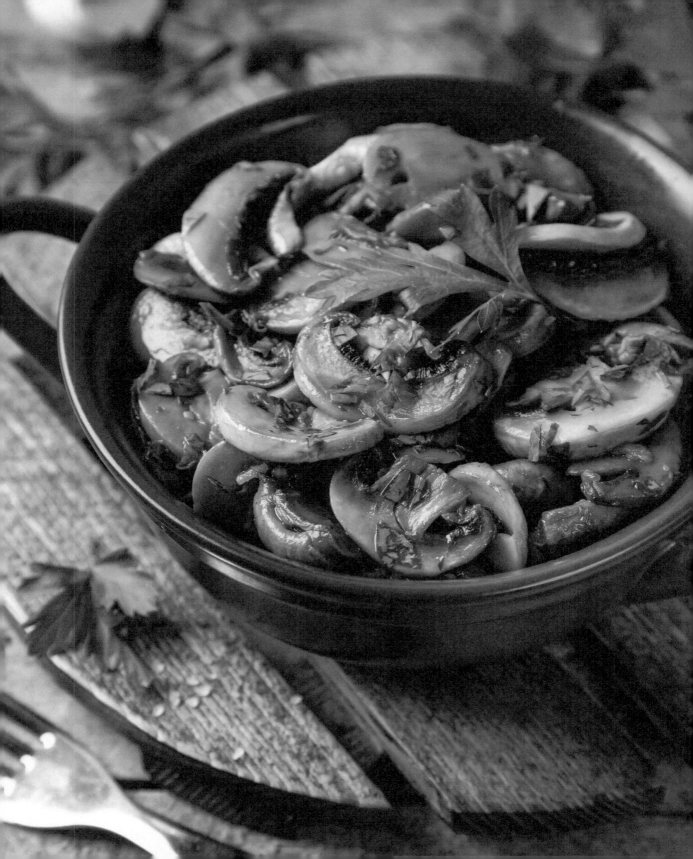

ZUCCHINI DIP

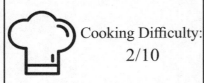 Cooking Difficulty: 2/10

 Cooking Time: 12 minutes

 Servings: 4

INGREDIENTS

- 2 spring onions, chopped
- ¼ c. veggie stock
- 2 garlic cloves, minced
- 2 zucchinis, chopped
- 1 tbsp. olive oil
- ½ c. yogurt
- 1 tbsp. dill, chopped

DESCRIPTION

STEP 1
Heat up a pan with the oil over medium heat, add the onions and garlic, stir and sauté for 3 minutes.

STEP 2
Add the zucchinis and the other ingredients except the yogurt, toss, cook for 7 minutes more and take off the heat.

STEP 3
Add the yogurt, blend using an immersion blender, divide into bowls, and serve.

NUTRITIONAL INFORMATION

Calories 76, Fat 4.1, Carbs 7.2, Protein 3.4

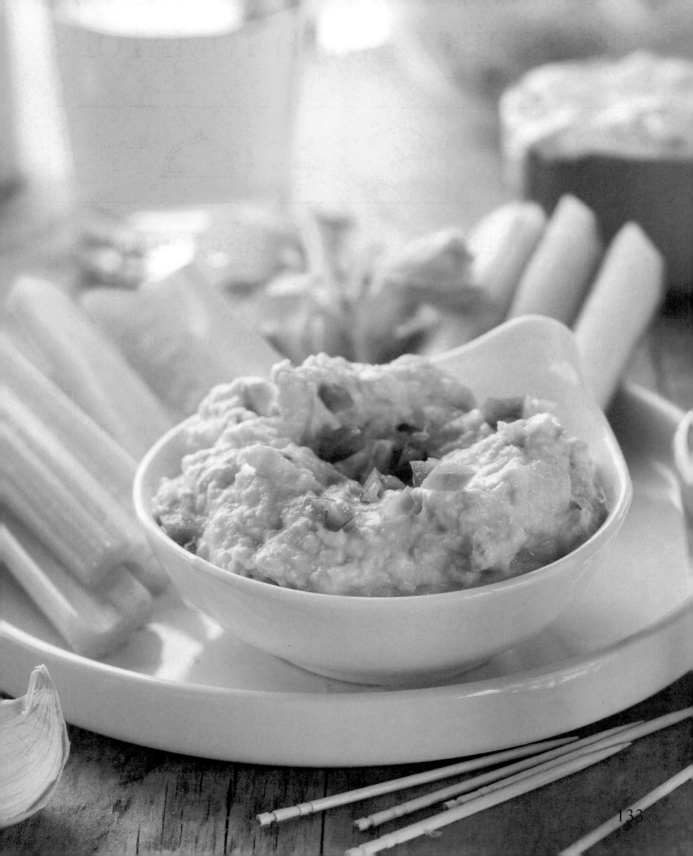

BRUSCHETTA WITH TOMATOES

 Cooking Difficulty:
2/10

 Cooking Time:
4 minutes

 Servings:
2

INGREDIENTS

- 1 sliced into thin pieces whole grain baguette
- 2 finely diced tomatoes
- 1 clove minced garlic
- fresh basil
- 2 tablespoons olive oil
- salt and pepper

DESCRIPTION

STEP 1
Toast slices of whole grain baguette in a dry skillet until golden brown.

STEP 2
In a bowl, mix diced tomatoes, minced garlic, chopped basil, olive oil, salt, and pepper.

STEP 3
Spoon the tomato mixture onto the toasted whole grain baguette slices.

NUTRITIONAL INFORMATION

123 Calories, 7g Fat, 2g Carbs, 5g Protein

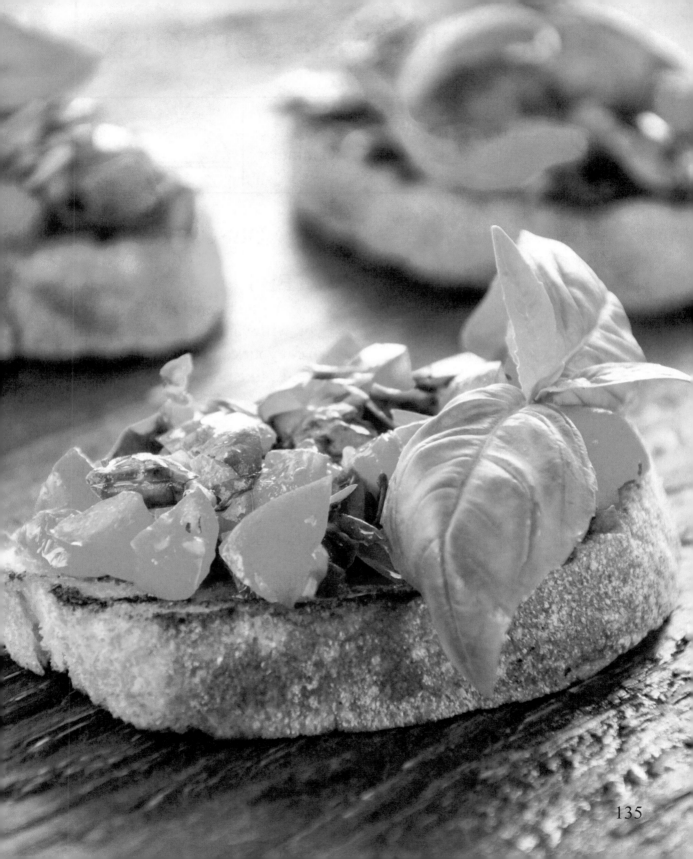

CAULIFLOWER POPCORN

Cooking Difficulty:
1/10

Cooking Time:
480 minutes

Servings:
4

INGREDIENTS

- 2 tbsps. olive oil
- 2 tsps. chili powder
- 1 tbsp. nutritional yeast
- 1 head cauliflower
- salt

DESCRIPTION

STEP 1
Before you begin making this recipe, you will want to take a few moments to cut your cauliflower into bite-sized pieces, like popcorn.

STEP 2
Once your cauliflower is set, place it into a mixing bowl and coat with the olive oil. Once coated properly, add in the nutritional yeast, salt, and the rest of the spices.

STEP 3
You can enjoy your snack immediately or place into a dehydrator at 115 for 8 hours. By doing this, it will make the cauliflower crispy! You can really enjoy it either way.

NUTRITIONAL INFORMATION

Calories: 100, Carbs: 10g, Fats: 5g, Proteins: 5g

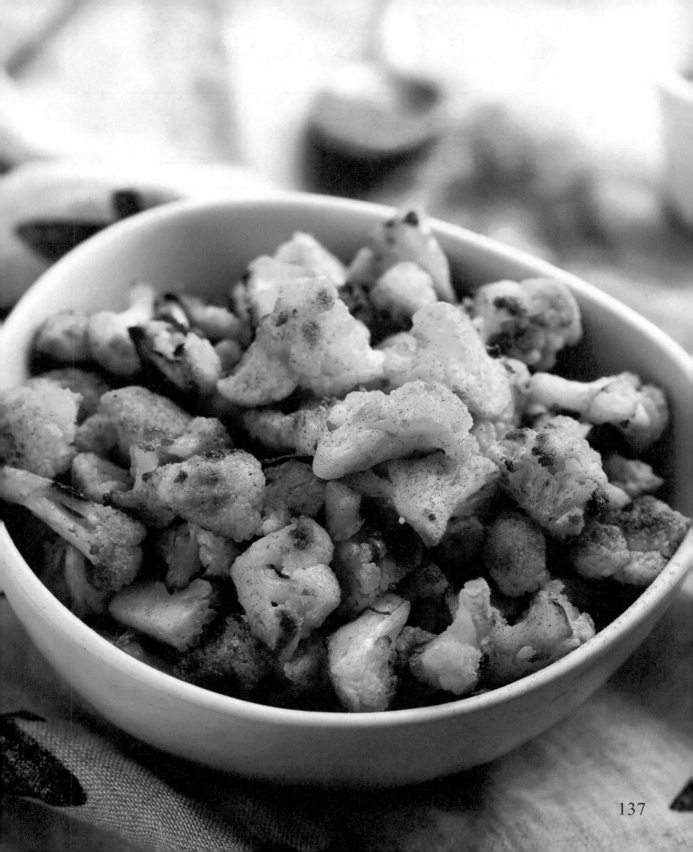

DELICIOUS HUMMUS

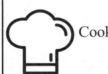 Cooking Difficulty: 1/10	Cooking Time: 4 minutes	Servings: 6

INGREDIENTS

- ¾ dried chickpeas
- 2 tbsps. olive oil
- 2/3 c. tahini paste
- juice of 2 lemons
- salt
- black pepper
- extra virgin olive oil for

  sprinkling

DESCRIPTION

STEP 1
Put the chickpeas in a large bowl with cold water and allow it to soak.

STEP 2
Drain and put in a saucepan with enough water to cover. Bring to a boil. Simmer on reduced heat for 1 hour, until chickpeas are soft and tender.

STEP 3
Transfer the chick-peas to a food processor and blend well to see a puree. Add in the olive oil, lemon juice, tahini paste. Mix well until smooth and consistent. Season with pepper and salt.

NUTRITIONAL INFORMATION

408 Calories, 23.6g Fats, 35.2g Net Carbs, 19.4g Protein

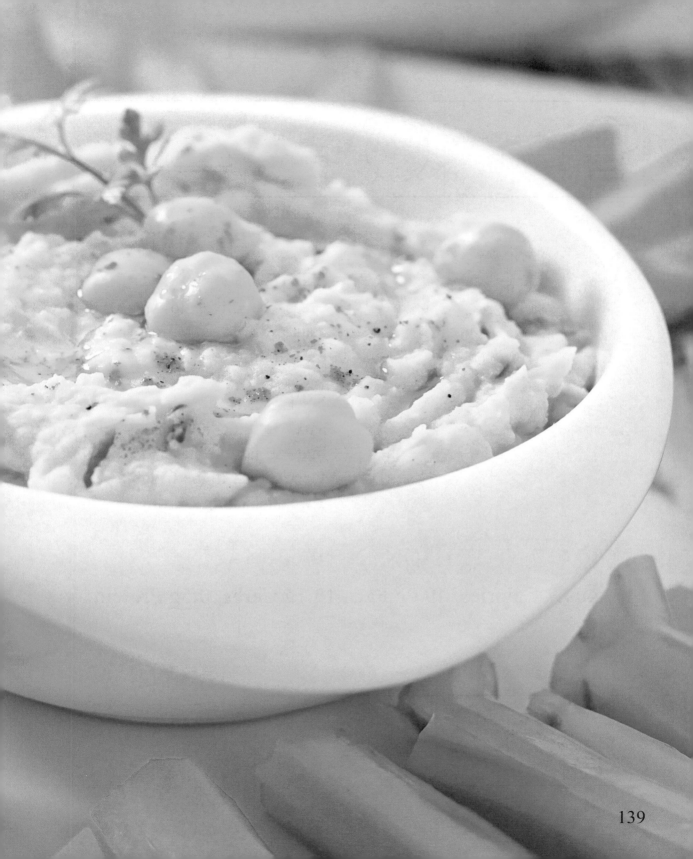

MARINATED OLIVES

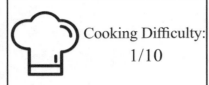 Cooking Difficulty: 1/10	Cooking Time: 2 minutes	Servings: 8

INGREDIENTS

- 1 1/3 c. green olives
- 4 tbsps. chopped coriander
- 1 crushed garlic clove
- 1 tsp. grated ginger
- 1 sliced red chili
- ¼ lemon

DESCRIPTION

STEP 1
Press the olives to break slightly, soak in cold water overnight, and then drain.

STEP 2
Mix well the ingredients and pour into the jars to marinade the olives. Place the jar in the fridge for at least 1 week, shaking 2-3 time.

NUTRITIONAL INFORMATION

404.7 Calories, 40.0g Fats, 13.1g Carbs, 0.5g Protein

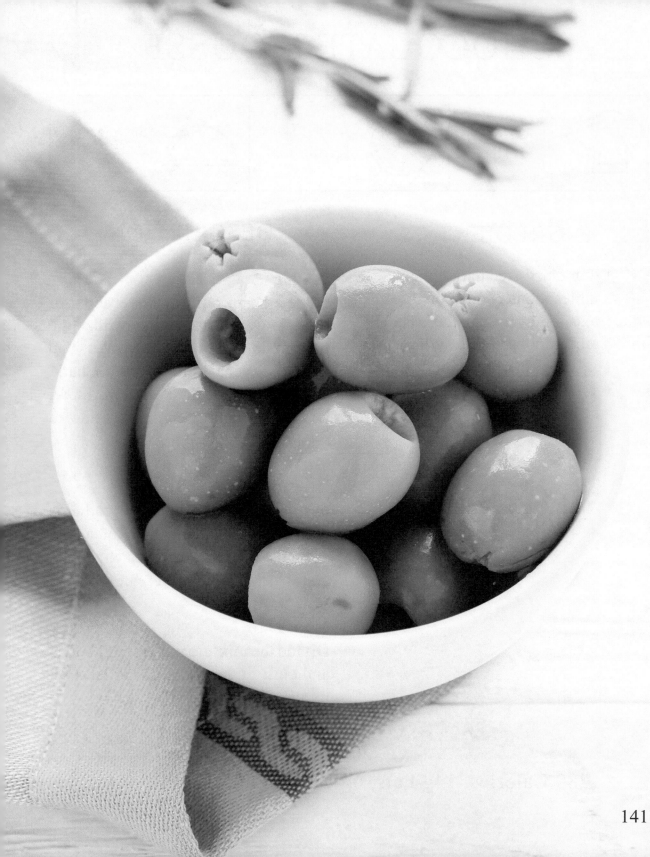

CHOCOLATE MOUSSE

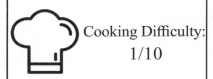 Cooking Difficulty:
1/10

 Cooking Time:
15 minutes

 Servings:
5

INGREDIENTS

- 170 g dairy-free dark chocolate
- 2 tablespoons cocoa powder
- 1 teaspoon vanilla bean paste
- 3 tablespoons maple syrup
- 1 x 160 g tin of coconut cream

DESCRIPTION

STEP 1
Place a heatproof bowl over a pot of boiling water, making sure that the bottom does not touch the water. You should have a kind of steam bath. Break the chocolate into the bowl and let it melt, then set it aside to cool slightly.

STEP 2
Pestle the remaining ingredients into the brander and mix for a few seconds. Pour in the cooled chocolate and whisk again until creamy.

STEP 3
Divide the mixture into 5 small bowls and chill in the fridge for at least 30 minutes. Serve.

NUTRITIONAL INFORMATION

280 Calories, 14g Fats, 6g Carbs, and 3,8g Protein

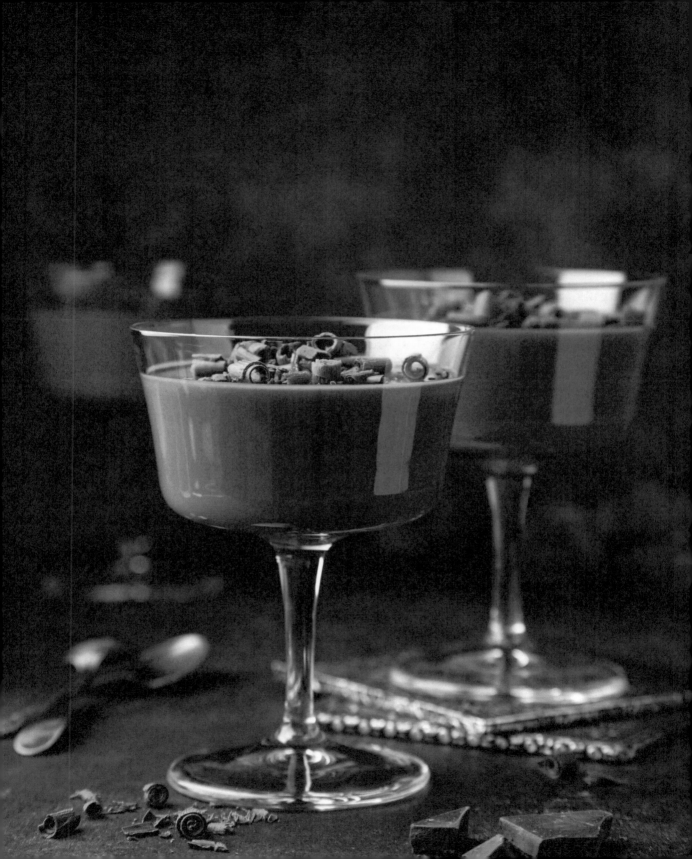

CONCLUSION

n conclusion, «MIND Diet: Brain Health Revolution» serves as a comprehensive guide to promoting brain health through mindful eating habits. Throughout this book, we've explored the intricate connection between nutrition and cognitive function, delving into the research-backed principles of the MIND diet.

By incorporating nutrient-rich foods such as fruits, vegetables, whole grains, lean proteins, and healthy fats into your diet, you can nourish your brain and reduce the risk of Alzheimer's disease and cognitive decline. The MIND diet emphasizes the consumption of foods rich in antioxidants, omega-3 fatty acids, vitamins, and minerals, which have been shown to support brain health and cognitive function.

Furthermore, we've provided a wide array of delicious and nutritious recipes that align with the principles of the MIND diet, making it easy and enjoyable to adopt brain-healthy eating habits. From vibrant salads and hearty soups to flavorful main dishes and satisfying snacks, these recipes offer a variety of options to suit every palate and dietary preference.

Incorporating the MIND diet principles into your lifestyle can have far-reaching benefits beyond just brain health, promoting overall well-being and longevity. By making small but meaningful changes to your diet and lifestyle, you can take proactive steps toward maintaining a sharp mind and vibrant cognitive function as you age.

As you embark on your journey to better brain health, remember that every food choice you make is an opportunity to nourish your body and mind. With the guidance and resources provided in this book, you have the tools and knowledge to make informed decisions that support lifelong brain health and vitality. Here's to a future filled with delicious meals, vibrant health, and a sharp mind!

Jerry Carr

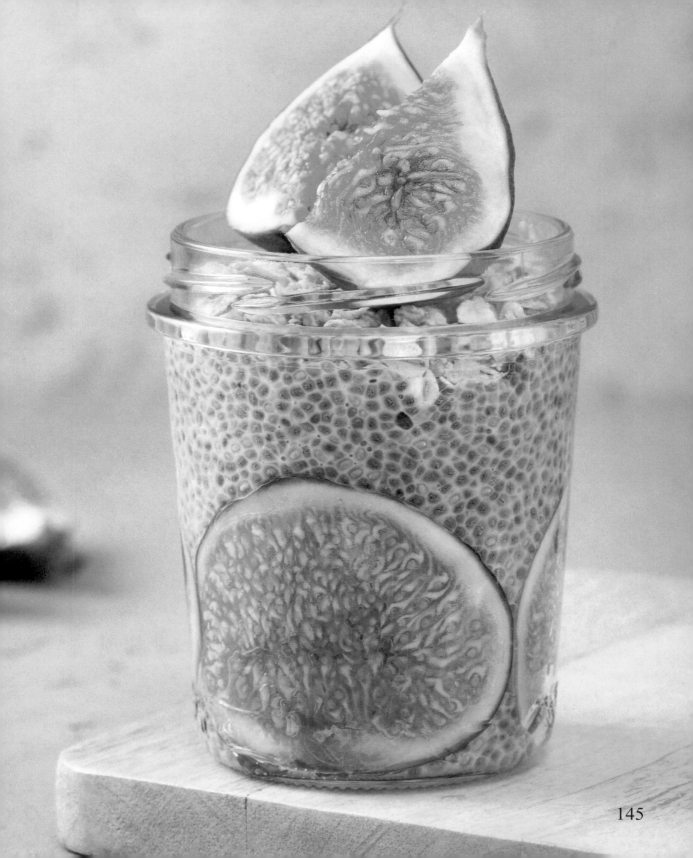

Made in United States
Troutdale, OR
07/06/2024

21053185R00082